THE ART OF
BLEPHAROPLASTY

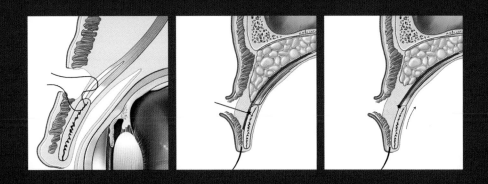

author **InChang Cho, MD PhD**

translator **Aram Harijan, MD**

군자출판사

THE ART OF **BLEPHAROPLASTY**

By Inchang Cho

1st Print : 2017-09-20
1st Publication : 2017-09-29

Translator : Aram Harijan
Publisher : Juyeun Chang
Editor : Eunhee Cho
Text Designer : Seonmi Park
Cover Designer : Sanghee Lee
Illustrator : Hohyeon Lee

Permissions may be sought at Koonja's rights department:
Tel: (82)-31-943-1888
Fax: (82)-31-955-9545
www.koonja.co.kr

Printed in South Korea
First Edition, © 2017 Koonja publishing, Inc.
ISBN 979-11-5955-234-2

THE ART OF
BLEPHAROPLASTY

About the author

- **EDUCATION**

1969-75	Medical School at Yonsei University (MD)
1978-83	Plastic and Reconstructive Surgery Residency at The Severance Hospital of the Yonsei University Health System
1984	Philosophy of Arts degree at Yonsei University (PhD)

- **EXPERIENCE**

1984	Plastic surgery fellowship at Keio University
1985-2011	Sole practice at Bando Eye Plastic Surgery Clinic
2006.10	International fellow at Paces Clinic in Atlanta, GA
2002-2004	President of the Korean Plastic Surgery Clinician's Association
2004-2006	President of the Korean Society of Aesthetic Plastic Surgeons
2000-	Clinical Professor of Plastic Surgery at Yonsei University
2012-	Partner practitioner at Bio Plastic Surgery

- **JOURNAL ARTICLES**

  Clinical Studies of Blepharoptosis. Archives of Plastic Surgery 1980;7:253-7 [in Korean]

  Early Revisoion of Unfavorable Upper Blepharoplasty. Archives of Aesthetic Plastic Surgery 2006;12:119-24 [in Korean]

  Treatment of Lower Eyelid Retraction. Archives of Aesthetic Plastic Surgery 2007;13:117-25 [in Korean]

  Surgical Correction of Multiple Upper Eyelid Folds in East Asians. Plastic Reconstructive Surgery 2011;127:1323-31

  Correcting upper eyelid retraction by means of pretarsal levator lengthening for complications following ptosis surgery. Plastic Reconstructive Surgery 2017;130:73-81

- **BOOKS**

  Oculoplastic surgery: Etiology and management of Complications following Double Eyelid
  Surgery. [in Korean]
  Asian Facial Cosmetic Surgery : Revision Double Eyelid Operation

Preface

Plastic surgery is a medical specialty founded on functional needs but, at the same time, has aesthetics as the primary goal. As such, outcomes within the discipline are subjective and varied according to individual tastes. This is how plastic surgery communicates with the Art.

From the beginning of my career, the given advice had been that oculoplasty is a difficult subject matter - a truth which became increasingly familiar with each subsequent year of practice. Outcomes once considered satisfactory decades ago are now considered wholly inadequate. The ever-increasing standard of beauty has become an unending demand, and technical completeness remains an elusive destination.

While the following is applicable to all of plastic surgery, outcomes in oculoplasty are especially sensitive to minor technical differences, which are both delicately sophisticated and sophisticatedly delicate.

A book is an incomplete medium for transferring knowledge; words, photographs, and illustrations can never adequately delineate subtle yet discrete details so important in blepharoplasty. From the eastern side of the Pacific Ocean, those of us practicing oculoplasty have strongly felt that pre-existing texts and body of literature have failed us. Faithfully, we have carried out operations as described and have learned of the painful consequence of blindly following the beaten path - not recognizing that we were exploring in an uncharted territory.

The book was prepared from the experiences I have gathered through a small practice in Seoul. There is a limit as to how much a single person's experience can be considered as a representative experience for others, and I consider my own experiences to be limited as such. Likewise, I do not suggest that a single chapter herein describes a superior version of oculoplasty. I do, however, believe in the philosophy which argues that explicit expressions of opinions become stepping stones for turning ethereal speculations into tangible hypotheses. Through expressing my dimly-lit opinions, the intention has been to solicit a brighter insight from truth-holders. It is my hope that others, whom with a different set of experiences and knowledge, will kindly point out to me the things I could have done better.

The book does not encompass the full spectrum of oculoplasty. Instead, its focus is on matters which are little discussed, varied in opinion, require extra emphasis, and/or have high potential for complications. Many readers will find that certain proven operations and techniques are missing. For these, I felt that my experiences were too limited to provide any opinion of value. In addition, there are details which are described repeatedly. The redundancy exists not to pad the page count but to provide the context wherever it is necessary for understanding the immediate sequence of ideas.

My hope is that the book guides the uninitiated away from those painful lessons I have learned the hard way. If it becomes a small context in the history of plastic surgery, it will happen because I was practicing where the part of history was happening at the turn of 20th century. If something in the book makes the reader smile and say, "Yeah, I made the same mistake, too", I would find solace in knowing that I was not alone in this remote wilderness these past twenty/thirty years.

I would like to extend my gratitude to my parents and my wife for the encouragement and inspiration. The preparation of this book would not have been possible had it not been for Mrs. Jisook Park's managerial role in overseeing the project. I also would like to thank the folks over at Koonja Publishing Company for the support over the years. Last but not least, I would like to express my endless gratitude to Dr. Jae Duk Lew, my teachers in plastic surgery, and collaegues who have provided the inspiring discussion over the years.

Sincerely,

In-Chang Cho, M.D.

Translator's foreword

If you are reading these words, then the translation project is complete. All the illustrations and page layouts have been finalized and approved. The book is out of the press, bound in the hardcover, and now, in your hands.

Perhaps you are holding this book first time at a plastic surgery conference wondering if you should take the book home. If this is the case, I can tell you that this book covers the subject matter of the book title exactly and that there is no other text that better covers this topic.

Perhaps this book is your own copy and you have read it over many times. In this case, you are most likely wanting to understand more than just the content of the book. You are probably looking for the context, in which the English version of this book came to existence.

To plastic surgeons in East Asia, Dr. Cho does not require an introduction. This being an English text, I imagine many readers will be unfamiliar with Dr. Cho's accomplishments in advancing the practice of blepharoplasty, especially in the management of severe congenital ptosis as well as complications of blepharoplasty operations.

As with all accomplished surgeons and artists, Dr. Cho is a person of singular focus. Observing him, I have often heard him mutter, "Have I have finished the task at hand? What else can I do to occupy this newfound time?" In all of the time I have observed Dr. Cho, I do not recall a single instance where he has shown some form of elation for having completed the task at hand, such is his drive to become a better artist and a surgeon.

I first met Dr. Cho back in October of 2009. I was a surgical intern at the UCSF-East Bay program in California, visiting Seoul for a short couple of weeks. I still vividly remember the conversation in which Dr. Cho explained the nature of scarring and how it is essential physiologic principle exploited in the surgical creation of supratarsal crease. I also recall the overflowing stacks and piles of articles and books on the desk of his private study within the clinic, all of which made apparent his immense desire to understand and improve the practice of blepharoplasty.

A few years rolled by. It was in December of 2014, when Dr. Cho called to ask if I could be available for the translation project. Very few people in the Western Hemisphere would understand the significance of this call, but to be offered the opportunity to translate the book was an opportunity of a lifetime. After all, there are plastic surgeons in remote parts of East Asia whose practices are built squarely on a mere photoshopped image of Dr. Cho.

The translation project began in early 2015 and took more than two years to complete. Rote translation of the Korean text into English proved to be impossible, as intricate descriptions of anatomy or surgical maneuvers did not easily yield to direct translations. Seeing the struggle, Dr. Cho provisioned an office for me within the clinic, from where I spent 3 months observing Dr. Cho and finally began to understand the Korean text. Much of this time with Dr. Cho is what is now reflected in this translated copy of the venerable surgeon's original text. It is my hope that the book portrays the Art of Blepharoplasty as faithfully as Dr. Cho originally intended in his native language and that the reader forgive me for poorly translated portions of the text.

Sincerely,

Aram Harijan, M.D.

Contents

CHAPTER

01

DOUBLE EYELID OPERATION

THE ART OF BLEPHAROPLASTY

- Considerations before double eyelid operation
- Design of the upper eyelid crease
- Mechanism behind the eyelid crease
- Non-incision, incision, and excisional operations
- Soft tissue excision
- Depth of eyelid crease
- Classification of fixation techniques
- Knot tying
- Skin suture
- Miscellaneous issue

CONSIDERATIONS BEFORE DOUBLE EYELID OPERATION

Atraumatic technique represents the highest form of surgery

If the goals of operation can be achieved with or without a specific maneuver, that maneuver is unnecessary and should not be employed. While this may be stating the obvious, certain maneuvers are performed solely for the psychological well being of the operator with no benefit to the patient. Such actions represent not only wasted labor but also add scar tissue upon the operated tissue – both should be avoided. Plastic surgery is a creative discipline with a basis on anatomy and physiology, and all plastic surgery operations must follow the principles of the natural law (FIGURE 1-2).

The single most important determinant of success for blepharoplasty is the appreciation for beauty

The standard for beautiful eyes varies with locality, race, and time, as well as by individual aesthetics, preference, and value. The individual aesthetics has to be agreeable with objective and standard for societally acceptable beauty. While keeping the objective standard in mind, the role of plastic surgeon is to understand a patient's desire for individual beauty, to provide the necessary medical knowledge, to guide the patient to a safe but desirable destination. Therefore, a one-size-fits-all approach to beautiful eyes is wholly inadequate for successful blepharoplasty. To develop the proper appreciation for beauty, an operator must be able to decipher the subtleties of a patient's eyes and their relationship to the rest of the face, all the while keeping in mind the patient's age, preference, and social context in which the patient must continue to interact.

A suture tension can never be the permanent source of fixation

When two tissues are brought together, adhesion is what eventually keeps these tissues from separating apart. During the few weeks following an operation, tissues stay in the new anatomic arrangement because of the tension provided by the sutures. In the case of eyelids, the repetitive force of blinking and the force of gravity loosen the tissue around the suture, and the surgeon must operate while keeping in mind that the sutures will not contribute to the fixation force after several months.

The risk of suture failure is greater for operations involving mobile or tensile tissues (i.e. correction of retraction and severe ptosis), and these require secure sutures with overcorrection of the eyelid margin. Also, adhesions form only between two immediately adjacent tissues. Fixations to hard tissues such as bone or tarsal plate will not form secure and direct adhesions if the contact surfaces are interposed with fatty tissue, which would prevent direct contact between the intended tissues. Such fixations would not be secure and can loosen over time.

Early recovery

People who are contemplating blepharoplasty are interested in minimizing the amount of time required for recovery – the time required to return to work and social functions. Many are deterred from undergoing blepharoplasty because they fear that recovery from the operation may take up to a year. How can this recovery time be shortened? The truth is that the rate for recovery is proportional to the simplicity of the operation. Recovery can be defined by the amount of soft-tissue change, with early recovery marked by minimal change in the tissue. For example, an operator may decide to perform an operation that creates a deep crease to overcorrect for significant loosening with postoperative changes. This will result in a longer period of recovery than an operation that creates a shallower crease anticipating less loosening of fold. Additionally, recovery time can be decreased via medical and physical means. Reduction in the time required for recovery requires a constant and concerted effort from both the operator and the patient.

The double eyelid

A person with natural double eyelid appears alert, approachable, and expressive. However, a botched double eyelid can appear wild and unnatural, as well as mistaken as an expression of discontentment or disapproval.

Double eyelid operation is indicated for eyelids that cause the appearance of sleepiness, piercing gaze, inexpressiveness, or timidity. Double eyelid appears the most natural in patients with thin eyelid skin and wide palpebral fissure. In such patients, the high crease design results in a relatively low eyelid crease that appears natural. In contrast, the eyelid crease can be designed relatively high yet still result in a crease that appears higher than intended, which makes the lower portion of eyelid appear thick and unnatural. In these patients, the operator should recommend a very minimal double eyelid operation.

Does double fold operation change the height of palpebral fissure?

The external visibility of an eyeball (pupil, iris, and sclera) is determined by the size of the palpebral fissure and the amount of eyelid skin drooping over the upper eyelid margin. Compared to a window, window size is determined by actual window size and the amount of blind covering the window. An eyelid with crease will display the entire palpebral fissure, whereas an eyelid without crease will mask the upper border of the palpebral fissure with the eyelid skin. Such phenomenon is referred to as pseudoptosis.

Double eyelid operation is raises the skin, which fully exposes the palpebral fissure and makes the eyes appear larger. The extent to which double eyelid operation increases the visible portion of the eye is therefore dependent on how much of the upper eyelid skin had previously covered the palpebral fissure (FIGURE 1-1).

In addition to the skin, one must consider whether double eyelid surgery can actually alter the vertical distance (i.e. height) of the palpebral fissure. In persons with normal upper eyelid function, double eyelid operation would not lead to significant changes in eyelid height. However, the operation can lead to noticeable decrease in the palpebral fissure height in patients with pre-existing but undiagnosed weakness of the upper eyelid levator. This decrease in eyelid height is accentuated for high eyelid crease. The change can be evaluated in the intraoperative setting. Provided that the upper eyelid margins are symmetric to begin with, creation of eyelid crease can lead to decreased eyelid height in the operated eye, compared to the height of the contralateral yet-to-be operated eye. The author has seen changes in eyelid height between 0 and -1.5 mm with oculi muscle to tarsal fixation. At times, patients do complain of decrease in palpebral fissure height after the operation. Such changes are extremely minor in patients with adequately functioning levator muscle but can be significant in patients with weak levator function. There are two potential causes for this phenomenon. One cause is that the levator muscles may have been under greater amount of contraction while the upper portion of the palpebral fissure was covered with the eyelid skin and is no longer compensating with the double eyelid operation. The other cause is that the slight change in the upper eyelid does not affect a healthy levator muscle but over-burdens the weak levator muscle.

In contrast to the decrease in palpebral fissure, double eyelid operation can actually lead to increase in the palpebral fissure height. This is caused by the decreased weight of the upper eyelid by the excision of soft tissue. A corollary can be drawn in patients who have lost weight (i.e. lighter upper eyelid) and have found that their eyes appear larger.

KEYPOINT

Changes in palpebral fissure size after double eyelid operation

Larger palpebral fissure
- The drooping eyelid skin has been elevated.
- The upper eyelid is lighter from excision of soft tissue.

Smaller palpebral fissure
- The oculi muscle to tarsal fixation has lead to increased physical load on the levator muscle.
- The compensating effort has been removed.
- Decreased eyebrow height and disappearance of levator compensation.

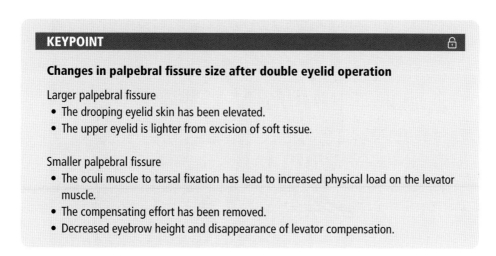
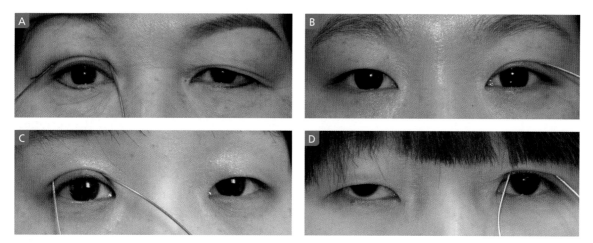

FIGURE 1-1 • Change in palpebral fissure after double eyelid operation.
The amount of pre-existing skin drooping determines the degree of change to the upper eyelid height.

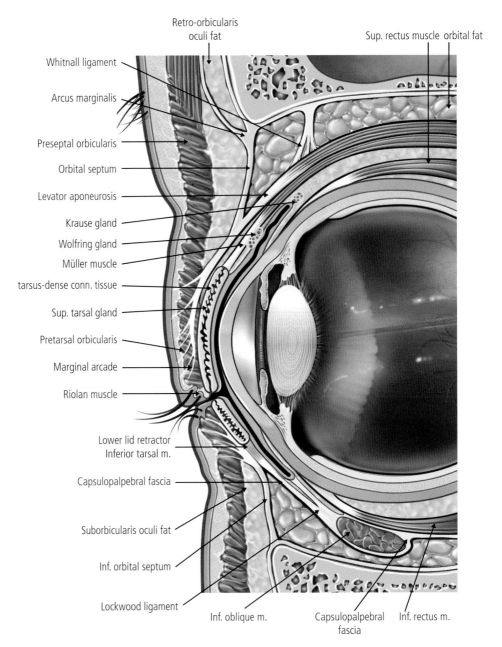

Retro-orbicularis oculi fat

Sup. rectus muscle orbital fat

Whitnall ligament

Arcus marginalis

Preseptal orbicularis

Orbital septum

Levator aponeurosis

Krause gland

Wolfring gland

Müller muscle

tarsus-dense conn. tissue

Sup. tarsal gland

Pretarsal orbicularis

Marginal arcade

Riolan muscle

Lower lid retractor
Inferior tarsal m.

Capsulopalpebral fascia

Suborbicularis oculi fat

Inf. orbital septum

Lockwood ligament

Inf. oblique m.

Capsulopalpebral fascia

Inf. rectus m.

FIGURE 1-2 • Anatomy of the eyelid (from Kang JS).

DESIGN OF THE UPPER EYELID CREASE

The upper eyelid crease must be designed with the patient in the upright sitting position. The height and shape of the crease are determined by various factors and must be considered in the design of the crease. The postoperative shape of the crease can be simulated using an eyelid stylus with the patient in the sitting position and demonstrated to the patient with a mirror. The process of determining the crease shape is an iterative process that requires conversation with the patient.

Blepharoptosis or blepharochalasia cannot be evaluated in the supine position. Also, the height of the eyelid crease differs between sitting and supine position, and the amount of skin to be excised cannot be evaluated in the supine position. The height of eyelid crease changes with variations in the palpebral fissure height. Also, it can also be affected by the patient's physical position and mood, as well as the amount of ambient light. For an extreme example, a patient can be observed to have a larger eye (larger palpebral fissure) on the right side in the sitting position but have a large eye on the left side while supine. For these various reasons, the eyelid crease should be designed and evaluated in the sitting position.

Types of eyelid crease
Double eyelids can be classified by the curvature, height, and depth of the crease.

Classification by curvature
- Inside fold
- Outside fold
- Neutral fold

Upper eyelid crease can be divided as being either inside or outside folds or as being either fan-shaped or parallel. Inside folds are fan-shaped, whereas outside folds can be either fan-shaped or parallel folds (FIGURE 1-3).

Inside fold
At the medial epicanthus, the inside fold is hidden inside the eyelid margin and grows wider towards the lateral epicanthus, which is why all inside folds are fan

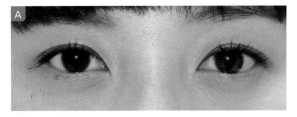
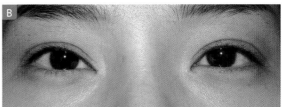
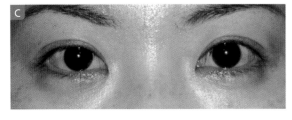

FIGURE 1-3 • **A.** Inside fold. **B.** Outside fold. **C.** Neutral fold (Right eye), Hybrid of inside and neutral fold (Left eye).

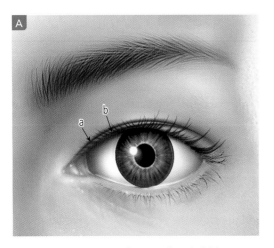
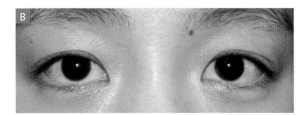
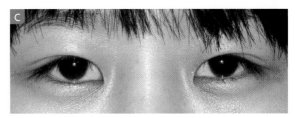

FIGURE 1-4 • Subclassification of inside fold.
A. These eyelid creases are subtle, nuanced, and natural.
    Line a: The eyelid margin intersects the eyelid crease medially. The look is elegant and sophisticated.
    Line b: The eyelid margin intersects the eyelid crease more laterally. Less of the palpebral fissure is visible.
B. These inside folds have long continuous margins. **C.** The insides folds are relatively short in this patient.

type folds. According to the beginning position, inside fold start medial or more lateral **(FIGURE 1-4)**.

Compared to outside fold, this type of eyelid crease does not lead to drastic changes in the appearance. It appears relatively natural but does not significantly increase the view of the eye (i.e. palpebral fissure) **(FIGURE 1-4)**. When the inside fold is desired by the patient, the author recommends creating the intersection between the eyelid margin and the crease as medially as possible (Line A), as it looks

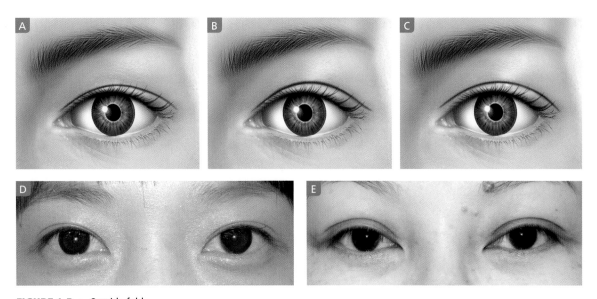

FIGURE 1-5 • Outside fold.
The crease should not be present for the 2-3 mm over the medial canthus.
A. Fan-shaped fold. The width of folds grows larger from medial to lateral eyelid. This is type of outside fold is possible for folds that are narrow overall. **B.** A combination of fan-shaped fold and parallel crease. The width between eyelid margin and crease grows from medial to central eyelid, at which point the crease follows a path parallel to the eyelid margin. This type of eyelid crease is most appropriate for normal eyelid fold. **C.** Parallel crease. The distance between the eyelid margin and crease remains the same over the whole length of the eyelid. This type of eyelid crease does not appear natural in East Asian patients. **D.** Left: The crease is narrow medially and becomes wider laterally. Right: The fold is neutral. **E.** Parallel crease with wide fold.

sophisticated and opens up more of the palpebral fissure.

Outside fold

An outside fold refers to upper eyelid creases which exists separately (i.e. does not intersect) from the upper eyelid margin. Outside folds can be fan-shaped, parallel, or a combination of the two. Fan-shaped folds are narrow medially and wider laterally **(FIGURE 1-5A)**. The outside folds with a combination of fan-shaped and parallel creases are narrow at the medial canthal region with creases that run parallel in the lateral portion of the eyelid **(FIGURE 1-5B)**. Parallel creases maintain an even, fixed distance to the upper eyelid margin from the medial to lateral canthus **(FIGURE 1-5C)**.

Outside folds are interpreted as elegant, expressive, and extroverted. However, such upper eyelid may betray the ethnic aesthetics of the patient and appear quite unnatural in Asian patients. Outside folds that are narrow medially appears elegant and expressive yet retain the naturalness of the inside folds. As such, the author frequently recommends elongated inside folds **(FIGURE 1-4A)** or narrow parallel outside folds (FIGURE 1-5B) to East Asian patients. It is better to create a discrete crease that begins 2-3 mm lateral to the medial canthus.

Neutral fold

This type of eyelid crease can be considered as an intermediate between the inside and outside fold. It has none of the disadvantages of inside or outside folds. It leads to relatively open view of the eyes while remaining natural.

Several factors should be considered in selecting the appropriate type of fold for a given patient. The first consideration is given to the canthal tilt. Fan-shaped fold works well with lower lateral canthus, whereas outside fold works well for patients with high lateral canthus. The second consideration should be made for the height of the eyelid crease. High creases tend to result in outside fold. Low creases tend to develop inside fold. Depending on the patient, however, such relationship may not be constant. If an upper eyelid with a tendency for inside fold is created into an outside fold, the medial portion of the crease will appear too high and unnatural. Patients with such eyelids should be steered away from receiving an outside fold. No eyelid crease that is higher medially can appear natural (FIGURE 1-6).

At times, patients may ask for the difficult combination of outside folds with low eyelid crease. This problem can be addressed through several means.

- The presence of epicanthal fold signifies a natural tendency for inside fold. Epicanthoplasty will remove this tendency.
- The incision should be extended further medially.
- The lateral portion of the incision should be made as low as possible. This has the effect of elevating the appearance of the medial slope and of the outside fold. The operator must be careful not to lower the incision too much, which can

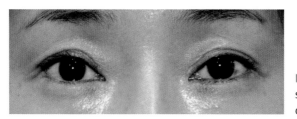

FIGURE 1-6 • The eyelid crease has a significant bend in the middle, and the crease is higher medially.

give the appearance of negative canthal tilt.

The decision between inside fold and outside fold is not always a dichotomous decision Generally, the author prefers inside and outside folds that closely resemble neutral folds.

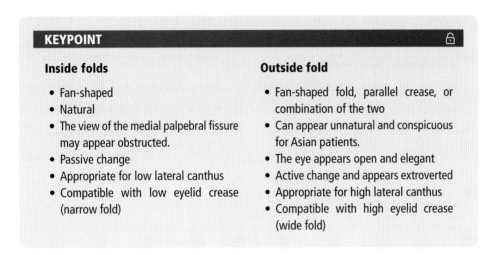

KEYPOINT

Inside folds

- Fan-shaped
- Natural
- The view of the medial palpebral fissure may appear obstructed.
- Passive change
- Appropriate for low lateral canthus
- Compatible with low eyelid crease (narrow fold)

Outside fold

- Fan-shaped fold, parallel crease, or combination of the two
- Can appear unnatural and conspicuous for Asian patients.
- The eye appears open and elegant
- Active change and appears extroverted
- Appropriate for high lateral canthus
- Compatible with high eyelid crease (wide fold)

The height of eyelid crease

A temporary eyelid crease should be created using a stylus with the patient in the sitting position. The height of eyelid crease should be selected only after a sufficient amount of discussion. The following should be considered in determining the appropriate height of eyelid crease.

- Large folds (large distance between eyelid margin and crease) are compatible with thin skin and large palpebral fissure. Small folds appear more natural for thicker skin and smaller palpebral fissure.
- Recovery time is proportional to the fold size. Larger folds tend to require longer recovery time with smaller folds resulting in quicker recovery. On the topic of recovery time, the author suggests that, in order for a postoperative eyelid to appear natural, recovery will take 1 week for small fold, 1-2 months for moderately-sized fold, and 4-5 months for large fold.
- One disadvantage of small fold is that the skin above the crease can sag over the years. The eyelid does not sag as much for larger folds. A good example of this is

Pablo Picasso, who does not demonstrate any dermatochalasis even in the 9th decade of life.

- The single biggest problem with larger folds is the hypertrophy of pretarsal area, which is described as "sausage eyes" among Korean patients. This is less of a problem for patients who have thinner eyelid skin and do not have as much pretarsal soft tissue, but represents a significant challenge for patients with thick pretarsal tissue who wish for large folds. Such patients should be counseled against having too large of eyelid folds for this reason. (Refer to the section on pretarsal hypertrophy in Chapter 3.)

- During the preoperative visit, patients view their own eyelids through the mirror. It is natural for most people to open their eyes slightly wider while viewing themselves through the mirror. This leads to an elevation of the eyelid margin by 0.5 to 1.0 mm, which conversely decreases the size of the fold. Thus, any crease designed while a patient is looking at the mirror can result in a larger-than-expected eyelid fold after the operation. For this reason, it is necessary to evaluate the eyelid fold that was designed while the upper eyelid was in a neutral primary gaze.

The double fold design requires evaluation of both patient factors and surgical factors. The patient factors are as follows.

- Skin thickness
- Skin laxity
- The amount of subcutaneous tissue
- Brow ptosis
- Levator function
- Hollowness of eyelid

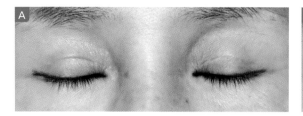 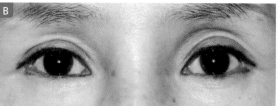

FIGURE 1-7 • With eyes closed, the eyelid crease appears to be higher on the right side. With the eyes open, however, the left eyelid crease appears to be higher because of the hollowness of the eyelid.

The fold becomes thicker if the skin or the subcutaneous tissue below the crease is thick. The fold becomes smaller if the skin is very lax or there is a severe ptosis of the eyebrows. Conversely, sunken eyelid offsets the laxity of the eyelid skin and increases the fold size (FIGURE 1-7). Thinner eyelid skin tends to contract under its own elasticity, which has the effect of decreasing fold size. The fold is also smaller for patients with powerful levator function.

If the skin is relatively taut, a stylus can be used to simulate the desired size of fold. However, laxity of skin will prevent accurate assessment. In such a case, an assistant can elevate the eyelid to simulate skin excision while the eyelid crease is designed. The brow should be elevated such that the eyelid skin should be stretched to 80-90% of the full length. (Refer to section on aging blepharoplasty in Chapter 2.)

The surgical factors that influence the fold size are as follows.
- Height of the design
- Depth of fixation
- Amount of skin excision
- Degree of ptosis correction
- Excision of periorbital fat

This topic will be discussed further in Chapter 3.

MECHANISM BEHIND THE EYELID CREASE

The eyelid is composed of
Anterior lamella – skin, subcutaneous fat, orbicularis oculi muscle layer
Middle lamella – orbital septum, orbital fat layer
Posterior lamella – levator aponeurosis, levator muscle, Müller's muscle,
tarsal plate, conjunctiva layer

The eyelid crease is connected to the levator aponeurosis between the anterior flap and the posterior lamella. When compared through electron microscopy, the difference between eyelids with and without eyelid crease can be appreciated in the expansions of the levator aponeurosis that penetrates through the orbicularis muscle (FIGURE 1-8). In creased eyelids, these penetrating branches connect to the dermis by a large number of septa found between the dermis and the orbicularis oculi muscle. In creaseless eyes, the aponeurosis does not pass through the orbicularis oculi muscle, or it penetrates the muscle too inferiorly (FIGURE 1-8). An eyelid crease can be created by the surgical formation of an adhesion between the anterior flap and the posterior flap.

The surgically created adhesions can be categorized as point adhesions, linear adhesions, or planar adhesions (FIGURE 1-9). The amount of adhesion is larger for linear adhesions compared to point adhesions, and in planar adhesions compared to linear adhesions. Because the tension is distributed through a wider contact, the chance of loosening of the fold is lower for planar adhesion. For narrow contacts, the chance of shallow fold is higher and in such cases overcorrections are necessary to accommodate for postoperative stretching. For this reason, point adhesions are appropriate for creating thinner eyelid folds, which are less likely to become undone.

Linear adhesions may be further categorized as partial and complete linear adhesions. In most cases, partial linear adhesions are at minimal risk of loosening of the fold, if the fixations were made securely. Compete linear adhesions are necessary in those cases where the chance of loosening is high.

The creation of planar adhesion is indicated only in special cases, as it is quite traumatic and may create too much scar tissue. As such, it is to be avoided except in extenuating circumstances. Planar adhesions are needed in the special case of failed crease operation, where the lower flap is severely adhered with scar tissue. In such a case, the lower flap should be adequately dissected, and the lower flap is redraped, which creates the planar adhesion between the anterior and posterior lamellae. (refer to p-104)

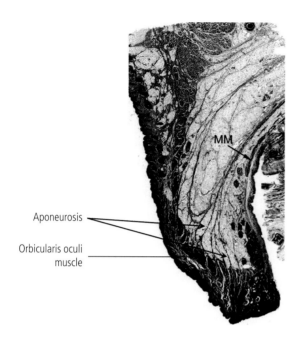

Aponeurosis

Orbicularis oculi
muscle

MM

FIGURE 1-8 ○ The levator aponeurosis penetrates the orbicularis oculi muscle and indirectly connects to the dermis, which creates the eyelid crease.
(photo from Department of Ophthalmology, College of Medicine, Donga University)
MM: Müller's muscle

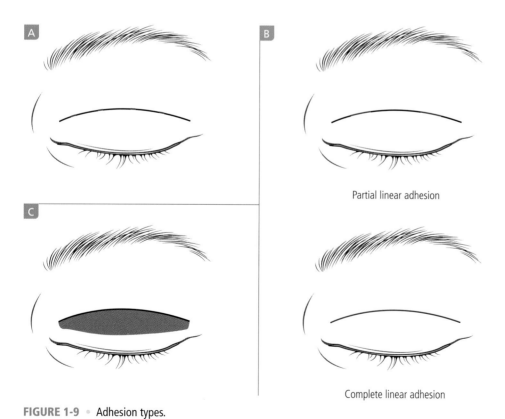

Partial linear adhesion

Complete linear adhesion

FIGURE 1-9 ○ Adhesion types.
A. Point adhesion. **B.** Linear adhesion. **C.** Planar adhesion. Red lines/area signifies adhesion between anterior and posterior lamellae.

NON-INCISION, INCISION, AND EXCISIONAL OPERATIONS

In elderly patients, the dermatochalasis requires skin excision. In younger patients, skin excision is required only for those patients with congenital excess of the eyelid skin. To evaluate whether skin excision is required, the patient is examined in the sitting position. A stylus is used to simulate the desired eyelid crease. If the elevation of eyelid demonstrates greater than 3 mm of skin drooping, the patient can benefit from skin excision. If there is not much skin drooping, the patient most likely will not benefit from skin excision (FIGURE 1-10).

Non-incision or short incision method

The non-incision method creates the eyelid crease without any soft tissue excision. The method creates minimal adhesion and is associated with high rates of failure. This method is most appropriate for thin eyelid skin with fine wrinkles and low resistance to crease formation. Non-incision methods tend to create adhesions that loosen after a period of time, so the creases should be made deep (ectropic).

Method I) Fixation through 3 stab incisions

Along the predetermined crease design, stab incisions (1-2 mm wide) are made at 3 points. The tarsal plate is fixated to the orbicularis oculi muscle below the skin

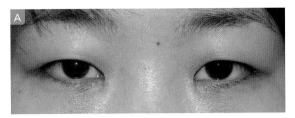
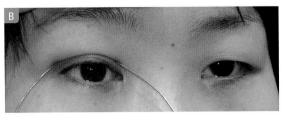
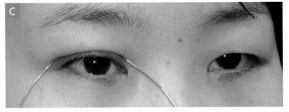

FIGURE 1-10 • **A.** Eyelids without crease. **B.** An assistant keep the eyebrow elevated while the eyelid crease is simulated. There is no significant skin drooping over the crease. **C.** The crease is simulated without elevating the eyebrow. There is significant skin covering the eyelid crease.

(FIGURE 1-11).

Method II) Fixation through 6 stab incisions

Along the predetermined crease design, six stab incisions are made in pairs at 5-6 mm intervals. The fixations are performed using 7-0 nylon double-arm sutures. One arm of the suture is introduced through the one opening, passed through the tarsus, and drawn out through the other opening. The other end of suture is inserted through the first opening, passed through the orbicularis oculi muscle, and withdrawn through the second opening. The loose ends are tied together. Two more sutures are placed in the same manner for the rest of the crease (FIGURE 1-12 & 1-13).

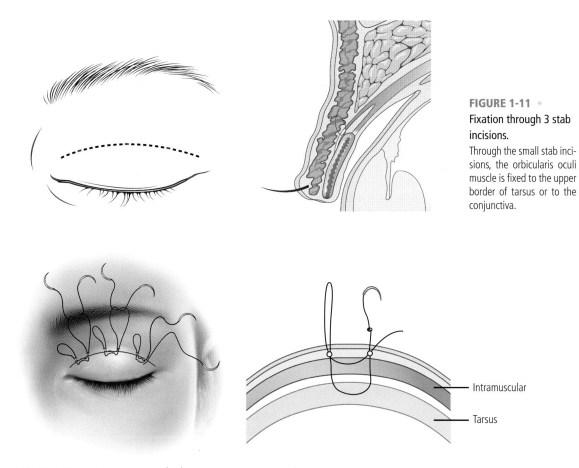

FIGURE 1-11 •
Fixation through 3 stab incisions.
Through the small stab incisions, the orbicularis oculi muscle is fixed to the upper border of tarsus or to the conjunctiva.

Intramuscular

Tarsus

FIGURE 1-12 • Non-incision method.
Three sutures are placed through 6 stab incisions.

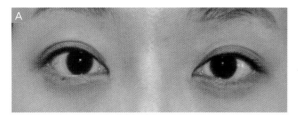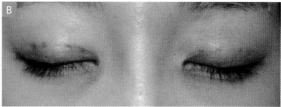

FIGURE 1-13 • This patient's eyelid creases were created through the 6 stab incisions.

Two partial incisions method

The author prefers this method, which utilizes a combination of stab incisions and small incisions. Like the non-incision method, the partial incision method has the advantages of minimal incisional scar, but it does not loosen easily as the partial incision access allows for excision of pretarsal tissue, which promotes strong tissue adhesion. Also, the short incisions are closed with eversion sutures to prevent the formation of depressed scars (FIGURE 1-15).

Indications

1. Younger patients
2. Eyelids without dermatochalasis
3. Eyelids with thin skin
4. Revision of low eyelid crease

When revising the low crease line to a higher location, the non-incision methods can be employed to prevention additional formation of scar tissue. In this case, the scar tissue in the lower flap can easily contribute to pretarsal bulkiness. To prevent this, the eyelid crease should not be made much higher than the crease from the primary operation. (Refer to the section on low eyelid crease in Chapter 3.)

Contraindications

- **Thick eyelid skin**: The partial incision approach is not appropriate when excision is necessary to reduce the bulk of retro-orbicularis oculi fat or the orbicularis muscle.
- **Loosened double eyelid crease with pretarsal adhesion**: The pretarsal adhesion interrupts the redraping of lower flap. This adhesion must be fully

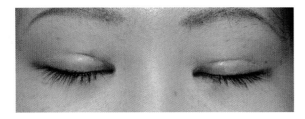

FIGURE 1-14 • Excision of orbicularis muscle has resulted in the depression scar along the blepharoplasty incision.

released prior to re-fixating the skin to the tarsal plate, which requires a full blepharoplasty access.

Operative detail

1. Two 4-mm incisions are made using a No.11 blade with stab incisions made on 2-3 mm away from the partial incisions.

2. Through the partial incision, the orbicularis muscle is divided using electrocautery or scalpel. The dissection is carried down to the tarsal plate.

3. To promote the adhesion between anterior and posterior lamellae, the pretarsal soft tissue is excised without sacrificing any of the orbicularis muscle. The reason for preserving the orbicularis oculi muscle is to prevent depression scar along the incision line **(FIGURE 1-14)**. The author avoids fixation of tarsal plate directly to the skin. Instead, the fixation is created between the plate and the orbicularis muscle.

   At this time, an operator may be tempted to completely excise the pretarsal tissue to fully expose the tarsal plate and promote strong adhesion. This is not advisable, however, because dissection of such aggressive nature causes significant scarring, decreased blood flow, delayed healing, and prolonged edema. Leaving the pretarsal aponeurosis, fixation to the tarsal plate and the aponeurosis above is a much better option than complete excision of the pretarsal soft tissue.

4. The initial loop of the suture needle is passed through the tarsus and aponeurosis from both incision lines, and the needle is withdrawn through the stab incision. Then, the suture is again passed from the stab incision, through the orbicularis muscle, and out the partial incision. The suture ends are tied. The same fixation is performed for all 4 stab incisions. These four fixations end up being 10 mm apart from each other **(FIGURE 1-15K)**. One important technical

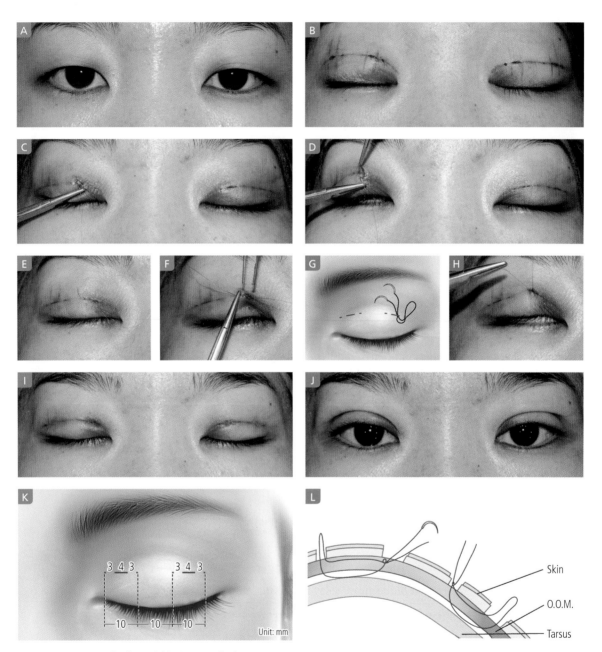

FIGURE 1-15 • Author's partial incision method.

A. Preoperative photograph. **B.** The crease design incorporates two 4-mm incisions with stab incisions on both sides. **C.** Through the partial incisions, the pretarsal connective tissue is excised. The initial loop of the suture is passed through the tarsal plate at the same level as the incision itself. **D.** The suture is then passed through the aponeurosis at a point 2 mm above the tarsal plate. **E.** The needle is withdrawn through the stab incision. **F.** The suture is pass from the stab incision, through the orbicularis muscle, and out the partial incision. **G.** Illustration of the fixation. **H.** The suture ends are tied. **I & J.** Postoperative photographs. **K.** The pattern of incisions. The 4 fixations are placed 10 mm apart. **L.** Cross sectional view of a fixation.

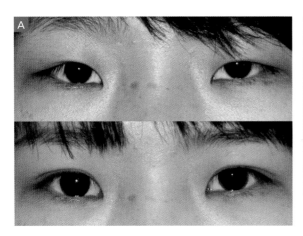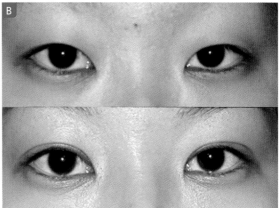

FIGURE 1-16 • These two patients underwent the partial incision method of eyelid crease formation.

detail is that the suture must be passed fully above and below the orbicularis muscle (subcutaneous and sub-orbicularis oculi plane) and that the suture knot must be buried deep to the orbicularis muscle. Details regarding fixation of the levator aponeurosis is discussed in the section for the advanced double fold method.

5. The skin is closed while incorporating the orbicularis muscle, which prevents the formation of depressed scar. The stab incisions do not need to be closed **(FIGURE 1-16)**.

Advantages of the partial incision method

1. Compared to open blepharoplasty, the method results in quicker recovery with less conspicuous scars.
2. The non-incision method tends to be loosened of the lack of adhesion formation, which is caused by the inability to excise the pretarsal tissue. This method allows the excision of pretarsal tissue and is less likely to fail because of the stronger adhesion.
3. The fixation incorporates a lot of the orbicularis muscle and is less likely to come loosened.
4. The incision is closed with everting suture, and the tarsal fixations are created under the stab incisions. These two factors significantly decrease the possibility of depressed scars.
5. The fixation points are evenly distributed every 8-10 mm.

The central incision method

Length of the incision

The incision does not need to be as long as the intended length of the crease. The reason for this is that, once the eyelid skin is forced to fold with tarsal fixation, the resulting crease tends to elongate in the axis perpendicular to the eyelid motion. Thus, a relatively short (10-12 mm) incision in the central portion of the eyelid may be sufficient in creating a crease that is much longer. However possible pitfalls should be understood.

Problems of central incision method

Shortness of crease

As mentioned above, a short incision can yield a full-length eyelid crease. However, this is not always the case, and the crease may not extend the full length of the eyelid if the skin is too thick.

Descent of the crease over the incision

The shape of the eyelid crease cannot be controlled beyond the points of fixation within the short incision. With a short central incision, it is possible for the crease to follow the shape of an outside fold. In Korean patients among whom epicanthal fold is common, there is a tendency for the tension of the epicanthal to bring down the crease into the shape of an inside fold (FIGURE 1-17). In such cases, central incision and fixation is inadequate, and the incision must be extended to control the shape of the crease. When the epicanthal fold is very defined, the incision may need to be extended as far medially as needed to maintain absolute control of the crease shape (FIGURE 1-18). Laterally, there is less of a tendency for the crease to descend. This is more common among elderly patients. In such cases, the incision should be extended laterally, and the crease should be fixated to the levator aponeurosis or the conjunctiva. (Refer to senile upper blepharoplasty in Chapter 2.)

Ideally, the lateral end of the crease should extend 4 mm beyond the lateral canthus (FIGURE 1-17).

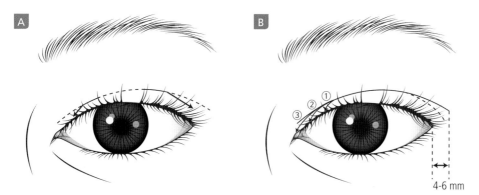

FIGURE 1-17 • **A.** The crease beyond the central area of fixation may descend. **B.** When the incision line is short with medial end at either Point ① or ②, the crease may not follow the intended line but curve towards the epicanthal fold. In such cases, the incision should be extended for the full length of intended crease.

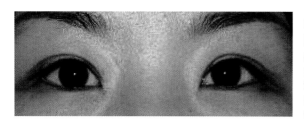

FIGURE 1-18 • In this patient, the left eyelid crease droops towards the epicanthal fold, causing an inside fold. If a patient wishes for an outside fold, the surgical incision should extend more medially to counteract the tension of the epicanthal fold on the eyelid skin.

The depth of eyelid crease

The eyelid crease can be deeply set at the incision site. At the same, it may be relatively shallow beyond the incision. This difference in depth can be highly conspicuous along the whole length of the crease. To minimize this contrast, the risk factors for depressed scar should be eliminated as much as possible. A depressed scar occurring only along a small central incision appears even worse than that of a full blepharoplasty incision. A detailed discussion of avoiding this problem can be found in the advanced blepharoplasty section.

The open blepharoplasty

The author limits the indication of open blepharoplasty to ① cases requiring excisions greater than 3 mm of skin and ② thick eyelids requiring removal of the orbicularis oculi muscle or the retro-orbicularis oculi fat. As a side note, simple orbital fat excisions can be performed via partial incisions.

Compared to open blepharoplasty, the non-incision method and short incision method are relatively simple operations with quicker recovery, less scarring, and natural appearance. However, these methods are not ideal even in younger patients if the upper eyelid is bulky and/or has redundancy of skin.

A common perception is that the non-incision method produces an eyelid crease that appears more natural than that created by open blepharoplasty. Most assume that this difference is a consequence of the incision itself. However, the author believe that the main reason open blepharoplasty produces unnatural eyelid creases is because of the extra maneuvers performed in open blepharoplasty that could not be performed during non-incision blepharoplasty. Such maneuvers include undermining and excessive removal of orbicularis oculi muscle of the lower flap causes significant scarring. If these maneuvers are avoided, open blepharoplasty can still result in an upper eyelid that is both beautiful and natural in appearance.

The advantage of open blepharoplasty is that it allows open access into the deeper structures of the eyelid and excision of redundant skin. It is indicated for dermatochalasis as well as patients who are beginning to show signs of periorbital aging.

In the author's experience, open blepharoplasty is required in approximately 20% of younger patients, but there is a wide spectrum of operator preference on this matter, as some excise a portion of the eyelid skin in all younger patients. The method of assessing skin redundancy will be discussed in Chapter 2.

SOFT TISSUE EXCISION

Orbicularis oculi muscle

The orbicularis oculi muscle does not need to be excised for non-incision and short incision blepharoplasty. The muscle should be excised, however, when accompanied by large amounts of skin excision in open blepharoplasty. If the orbicularis oculi muscle is removed in the absence of any skin excision, the resulting scar will be conspicuously depressed. Also, the author prefers to create the crease fixation between the tarsal plate and the orbicularis muscle instead of a direct connection between the plate and the skin. Because of this, it is best to minimize the excision of orbicularis muscle. The muscle may need to be excised if significant hypertrophy of orbicularis oculi muscle interferes with formation of crease. In such cases, the muscle is excised while preserving a cuff of the pretarsal orbicularis muscle. It is important to preserve this muscle near the incision line to minimize the risk of depressed scar.

Pretarsal soft tissue

Excision of pretarsal soft tissue promotes the adhesion between the anterior lamella (skin and orbicularis oculi muscle) and the posterior lamella (tarsus or levator aponeurosis). This is especially important if there is an excess of pretarsal fat in the medial eyelid, which can cause bulging and increase the likelihood of fixation failure.

One important aspect of pretarsal tissue excision is that the pretarsal tissue should be excised at a level inferior to the fixation sutures. In other words, the fixation sutures must be placed at the topmost edge of the pretarsal excision. If the fixation is performed in the central portion of the excised surface, an adhesion may form superiorly to the fixation, which can cause additional creases (AKA triple fold) **(FIGURE 1-19)**. (Refer to the section on triple fold in Chapter 3.)

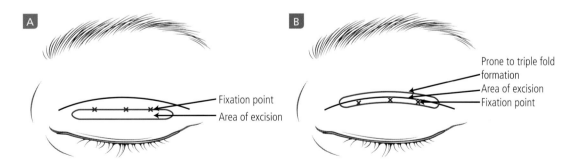

FIGURE 1-19 • Presence of excised surface superior to the tarsal fixation can lead to additional eyelid crease.
A. The fixation sutures are placed at the uppermost edge of the excision.
B. The fixation is performed through the center of the excised surface, which allows adhesions above the fixation line. This can lead to the formation of triple fold.

WAIT A MINUTE!

MANAGEMENT ON THE TARSAL PLATE IS SAFE

Soft tissue excision on the tarsal plate

The formation of eyelid crease is promoted by the excision of the connective tissue and the formation of adhesion. Thus, the excision must not extend beyond the upper border of tarsal plate. Excision of connective tissue superior to the tarsal plate is associated with the two following risks:

① Excision of tissue superior to tarsal plate can lead to inadvertent injury to the levator aponeurosis, which will lead to iatrogenic ptosis. The levator aponeurosis inserts into the border of tarsal plate by fibrous bands (**FIGURE 1-20**). Because of this fibrous connection, the levator mechanism is not interrupted by the excision of soft tissue that is anterior to the tarsal plate. However, excision of tissue superior to the tarsal plate can sever these connections. Disinsertion of the levator aponeurosis will be compensated by Müller's muscle for a time being, but will eventually lead to premature failure of the Müller's muscle, which ultimately leads to ptosis.

② Excision of connective tissue above the superior border of tarsal plate can lead to the formation of an additional adhesion between the anterior and posterior lamellae. This extra adhesion will then lead to the formation of an extra eyelid crease superior to the surgically created eyelid crease (i.e. formation of triple fold).

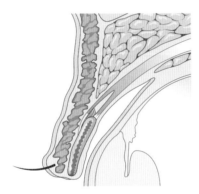

FIGURE 1-20 • Illustration of the fibrous bands connecting the levator aponeurosis to the superior border of the tarsal plate (red diagonal lines). A dense collection of fibrous bands form the connection between the levator aponeurosis and the tarsal plate. Excision of the soft tissue anterior to the tarsal plate does not affect these bands, but excision of soft tissue superior to the upper border of the tarsal plate may sever these bands and cause aponeurosis disinsertion.

Tarsal fixation (FIGURE 1-21)

If the fixation sutures are placed superior to the tarsal plate, the suture knots will not be isolated by the tarsal plate. Without the tarsal plate in the way, the suture knots can come into direct contact with the conjunctiva, which can cause irritation and pain. This is to be avoided especially for ptosis correction. Levator plication should be performed by fixating the levator aponeurosis to the tarsus such that the tarsal plate is interposed between the knot and the conjunctiva. If the plication is performed solely between two points of the levator, the suture knot may end up irritating the conjunctiva and the sclera.

Furthermore, the presence of suture knot is not safe even at the superior border of the tarsal plate, which may result in severe dimpling of the palpebral conjunctiva or irritation of the eye with each movement of the eyelid. As such, the suture must be placed within the top 1 mm of the upper tarsal border. Also, the sutures should partially penetrate the tarsal plate to withstand the tension of eyelid retraction. If the sutures do not penetrate the tarsal plate, the knot may migrate superiorly due to stretching of the tissue.

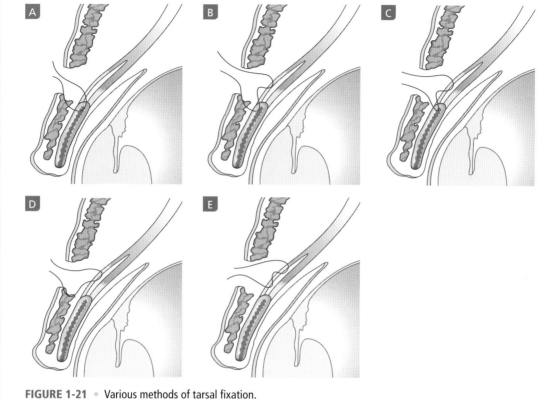

FIGURE 1-21 • Various methods of tarsal fixation.

Safe placement of the fixation knot over the tarsal plate:

A. Fixation of the flap to the tarsal plate.

B. Fixation of the flap and aponeurosis on the tarsal plate.

C. Fixation of the aponeurosis on the tarsal plate in levator aponeurosis advancement for ptosis correction.

Unsafe placement of the fixation knot superior to the tarsal plate:

D. Fixation of the flap to the aponeurosis.

E. Plication of the levator aponeurosis only results in a floating knot superior to the plate.

Orbital fat and retro-orbicularis oculi fat

In bulky upper eyelids, buttonhole incisions are made on the septum to remove orbital fat. The access through the septum does not need to be large, and large defects in orbital septum can cause unwanted adhesions which can lead to triple fold. Also, excessive excision of orbital fat should be avoided unless the upper eyelid is extremely bulky. One should remember that the volume of orbital fat decreases with aging.

If the excision of the orbital fat is insufficient, the upper eyelid bulk can be further reduced with the excision of retro-orbicularis oculi fat (ROOF). The ROOF is excised without exposing the periosteum, nor should the ROOF be excised near the orbicularis oculi muscle. Exposure of either the orbicularis muscle or the periosteum may cause adhesion and triple fold. Because the ROOF is superficial, even a small excision can cause significant surface irregularity. All of the potential complications of ROOF excision is compounded in the medial eyelid, where the ROOF is thinner. The ROOF lateral to the lateral end of eyelid crease should be preserved because removing too much ROOF from this location may lead to flattening of the lateral eye, which can give the appearance of cachexia and tiredness (**FIGURE 1-22**).

In contrast, the excision of soft tissue including oculi muscle should be limited to

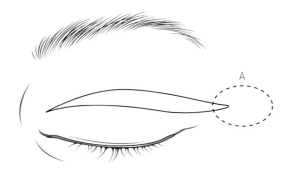

FIGURE 1-22 • Excision of the retro-orbicularis oculi fat in the lateral periorbital tissue, as shown by A, may cause the patient to appear cachectic.

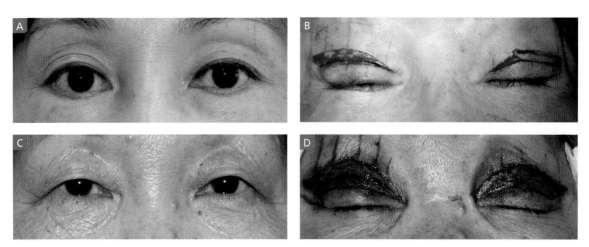

FIGURE 1-23 • In hollow eyelids, the connective tissue including orbicularis oculi muscle is not excised despite skin excision. The orbicularis oculi muscle is divided such that the extra tissue is used to bolster the flap that requires bulkiness.
A & B. The orbicularis oculi muscle is divided inferiorly to allow more of the muscle flap to be included in a superior flap with hollowness.
C & D. The orbicularis muscle can be divided evenly between the upper and lower flap.

skin excision, if the upper eyelid is thin or appears hollow. The muscle is to be used to add bulk to the thin eyelid **(FIGURE 1-23)**. Bulging medial fat should be excised and transposed as a free graft to a more lateral portion of the eyelid.

The author recommends against the undermining of lower flap or the excision of orbicularis oculi muscle on the lower flap. In most circumstances, the crease simulated by eyelid stylus can be obtained without the excision of the orbicularis oculi muscle and without depressed scars.

Other operators may advocate the dissection of the lower flap or excision of the orbicularis muscle from the lower flap for the following stated reasons.

Dissection into the lower flap helps to create adhesion for the eyelid crease

This is a reasonable argument. However, a securely created linear adhesion is just as effective at maintaining an eyelid crease. Also, the increase in adhesion from excess scar tissue is the exact reason an eyelid appears to have highly unnatural after multiple blepharoplasty. Because of the scar tissue, the skin loses much of its elasticity, and this interrupts to decrease the height of fold with elevation of eyelids. Setting aside exceptional situations, dissection of the lower flap should be avoided at all cost **(FIGURE 1-24)**.

Excision of orbicularis oculi muscle can prevent pretarsal hypertrophy

This is the most commonly used excuse for excision of pretarsal orbicularis muscle.

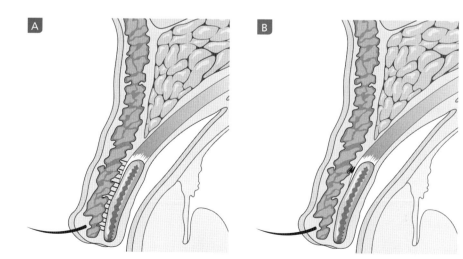

FIGURE 1-24 •
Comparison between planar adhesion (**A**) and linear adhesion (**B**).
In most situations, a secure linear adhesion is sufficient in maintaining an eyelid crease.

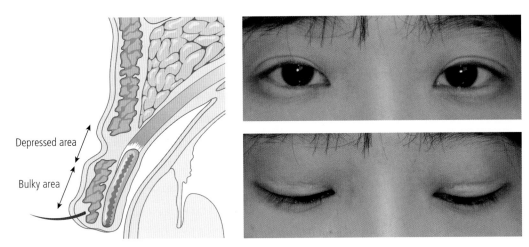

Depressed area

Bulky area

FIGURE 1-25 • Excision of orbicularis oculi muscle below the incision will create scar depression, along with the illusion of a relatively full pretarsal tissue. With the eyes closed, removal of orbicularis oculi muscle below the crease can be seen as the severe scar depression. With the eyes open, the visible portion of the pretarsal eyelid appears bulky.

In theory, excision of the pretarsal muscle should decrease the pretarsal volume, but this is not the case in practice. When the eyes are open, the eyelid crease is about 2-3 mm above the margin of upper eyelid. The lower 3 mm of pretarsal space is occupied by the marginal arterial arcade as well as the root of eyelashes. Thus, the orbicularis muscle is always excised above this initial 3 mm of the lower flap, causing an inadvertent contrast in the amount of pretarsal soft tissue that is appreciated as pretarsal hypertrophy while the eyes are open (**FIGURE 1-25**).

Other considerations in handling of soft tissue

In addition, dissection of the lower flap causes prolonged edema due to disruptions in the lymphatic and venous circulation. In severe cases, this can lead to chemosis. Another important complication arises from one of the functions of the pretarsal orbicularis muscle, which serves to pump and distribute tear with each blinking movement. As such, excision of this muscle can lead to a significant disability in the lacrimal function and the development of dry eye syndrome. The weakness in closing the eyes may contribute to nocturnal lagophthalmos. Even in the absence of lagophthalmos, weakness of the pretarsal muscle can lead to significant disabilities in the eyelid function.

Injection of botulinum toxin to the pretarsal oculi muscle elevates the upper eyelid margin. This phenomenon demonstrates the relationship between the pretarsal muscle and the height of palpebral fissure. Also, infiltration of local anesthesia into the pretarsal muscle can be observed in patients who experience temporary inability to close the eyelids fully. Both of these observations serve to highlight the importance of the pretarsal muscle in the closing the eyelids.

Another complication following excision of pretarsal orbicularis muscle is the development of telangiectasis of the eyelid. In such cases, the portion of the eyelid below the crease can appear dusky.

During the evaluation of an eyelid, the portion of the eyelid inferior to the simulated crease can appear too hypertrophied. In such a case, the hypertrophy should not be approached by the excision of the pretarsal soft tissue. Rather, this unwanted pretarsal fullness should be addressed by lowering the height of the eyelid crease. It is rare for the lower portion of upper eyelid to be bulky while the crease height is appropriate. If this is the case, however, a lower eyelid crease should be recommended to the patient.

DEPTH OF EYELID CREASE

Variations in the depth of eyelid crease/fold (FIGURE 1-26)

Shallow crease
- Characteristics and morphology are inbetween creaseless eyelids and eyelids with deep fold.
- Entropion
- Eye fissure is not completely exposed from the skin drooping

Moderate crease
Natural. This is associated with larger palpebral fissure.

Deep crease (fold)
- Ectropion
- Unnatural appearance

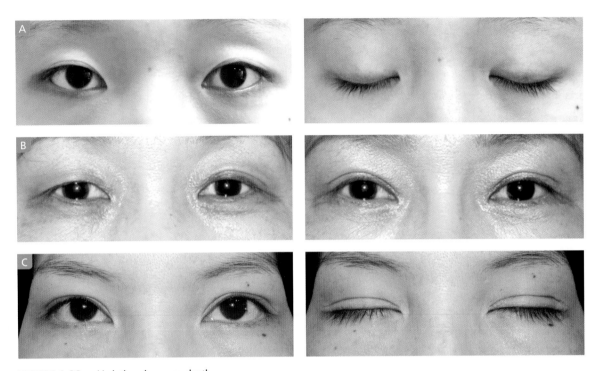

FIGURE 1-26 • Variations in crease depth.
A. Shallow crease. The true margin of the upper eyelid is covered by the skin over the eyelashes. **B.** Moderate crease. (Left) The left eye has a congenital crease; the right eye does not. (Right) After blepharoplasty of the right eye, the eyelid creases are symmetric. **C.** Deep fold. The eyelids have depressed scars and ectropion.

- Tugging sensation of the eyelid
- Depressed scars
- The eyelid appears bulky above the fold.
- The palpebral fissure is larger or smaller at times.
- Association with dry eye syndrome

In surgical creation of supratarsal fold, the opposite of ectropion is not entropion but shallow (faint) eyelid crease.

All eyelid creases become undone to a degree after a certain amount of time (FIGURE 1-27).

The depth of eyelid crease is the most important yet difficult problem to be solved. The shape and height of the crease are also important, but these can be evaluated during the preoperative examination, and as long as the fixation follows the

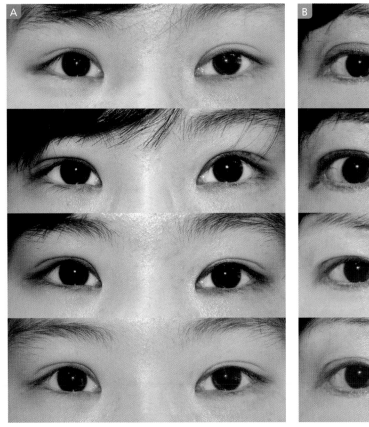 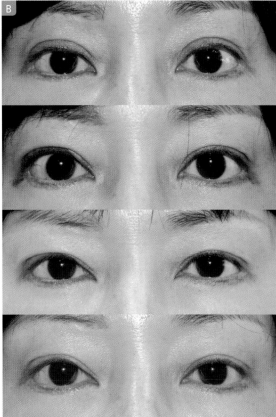

FIGURE 1-27 • Changes in eyelid folds over time.

A. Before operation

At 1 week, the upper eyelid creases are distinct.

At 3 months, the creases have become more faint.

At 8 months, the creases have faded significantly.

B. Before operation. The eyelids have ectropion.

At 10 days, the folds are slightly deep.

At 40 days, the folds are no longer deep.

At 6 months, the ectropion has resolved.

design, the shape of eyelid creases are relatively predictable. However, the crease depth can vary widely depending on patient factors as well as operative variations. The depth also changes with time, which makes it that much more difficult to communicate the expected outcome to the patient.

The degree to which the crease depth changes over time is dependent on two major factors. The first is related to the patient. There is a tendency for all objects to maintain its shape and to resist any force that attempts to change this shape. This can be thought of as a type of the moment of inertia, and can be applied to the upper eyelid. In eyelids with great resistance against crease formation, surgically created eyelid creases tend to are more likely to become fainter or become undone.

High resistance to crease formation can be expected for the following:

- Thick eyelid skin
- Severe dermatochalasis
- Hypertrophic soft tissue
- Weakness of levator muscle (ptosis)
- Tension in the medial skin from epicanthal folds
- Younger patients
- History of failed eyelid crease operation

The amount of resistance to eyelid crease can be observed by simulating the crease in the sitting position. Only a light touch of the stylus is required to simulate an eyelid crease for low-resistant eyelids, and the temporary crease tends to stay in place for a while. In contrast, the disappearance of crease as soon as the stylus is removed signifies great resistance.

Saggy skin covering the eyelashes

If the eyelid skin is lax enough to cover the base of eyelashes, the force required to create the eyelid crease must bear the weight of this skin. Simulation of the eyelid crease will reveal the amount of such force required. A great force required to simulate the crease signifies higher resistance of the eyelid to crease formation. In contrast, eyelids with low resistance tend to allow the creases to form with a light touch of the stylus (FIGURE 1-28B, 1-29).

Eyelids with weak levator function

Eyelid crease operations tend to fail in patients with weak levator function (i.e. ptosis) when the double fold operation is performed without ptosis correction. In such cases, the fixation should be performed to create deep folds. In contrast, such deep folds are not necessary if ptosis correction is performed concomitantly, as creation of deep fold can easily lead to ectropion. Even with ptosis correction, one should be aware of the fact that the lateral portion of the eyelid crease or fold can still become undone, where the levator aponeurosis is not advanced. To avoid this issue in the lateral eyelid, the author fixates the orbicularis oculi muscle to the tarsus and to the levator aponeurosis higher up (3-7 mm from the upper border of tarsal plate). (FIGURE 1-31, Refer to the section on ptosis in CHAPTER 5.)

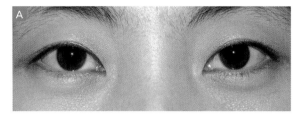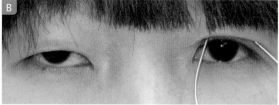

FIGURE 1-28 • **A.** Eyelids with thin skin are less likely to lead to a failed eyelid crease operation. **B.** Eyelids with skin covering the base of eyelashes are highly resistant to crease formation. Operative failures are more common.

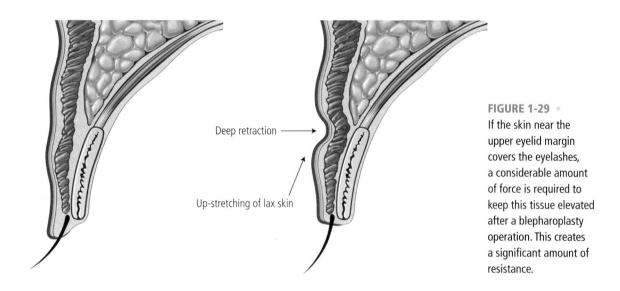

FIGURE 1-29 •
If the skin near the upper eyelid margin covers the eyelashes, a considerable amount of force is required to keep this tissue elevated after a blepharoplasty operation. This creates a significant amount of resistance.

Epicanthal fold

In eyelids with strong epicanthal bands, the stylus requires a significant amount of pressure against the medial eyelid skin to create an outside fold, which can be interpreted as large resistance in the medial eyelid. Releasing the epicanthal band can reduce the tension significantly. If an epicanthoplasty is not performed concomitantly, the fixation should be performed with the eyelid in a more ectropic position to avoid weakening of the crease.

Due to the tension on the skin from epicanthal fold, the medial side of the double fold often weakens when creating outside folds. However, this is not a problem for inside folds, which is not subjected to the tension of epicanthal fold **(FIGURE 1-30)**.

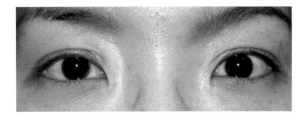

FIGURE 1-30 • Weakening of the medial eyelid crease due to epicanthal folds.
Creation of outside folds in eyelids with epicanthal folds often leads to failure of tarsal fixation in the medial portion.

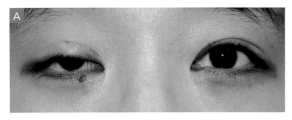

FIGURE 1-31 • The eyelid crease is much fainter from the ptosis.

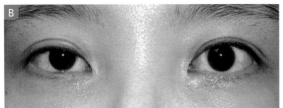

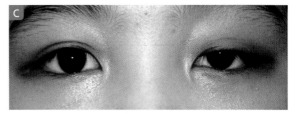

Patient age

Older patients tend to have eyelids with low resistance to crease formation, due skin laxity and decreased subcutaneous tissue. For this reason, eyelid crease operations tend to be deeper in the elderly population and are more likely to be faint in younger patients.. The crease should be made deeper than usual to promote slight ectropion because the crease will become shallower with time in younger patients.

Secondary operation

Among various predictors, the most likely cause of operative failure is prior history of crease operation failure. In such secondary cases, the prior operation has resulted in adhesion to the lower flap which hinders the redraping maneuver. If this lower flap adhesion is severe, the surgeon may not be able to simulate crease line with an eyelid stylus in the preoperative setting. If the adhesion is minor, the operation can proceed as usual, but if the adhesion is severe, the operation will be a challenging one. To create an outlasting crease in the presence of lower flap adhesion, the following procedures should be observed: ① the lower flap should be dissected to release the adhesions, which would allow the redraping of lower eyelid and ② the crease should be fixated higher than usual and slightly ectropic because the lower flap tissue is stiff from the remaining scar tissue. This is discussed in more detail in the complication of crease operation in Chapter 3.

Of the various causes for weakening of the creases, the most likely case for crease failure is the one with a combination of the risk factors mentioned above. For example, the chance of operative failure is extremely high in the case of an eyelid with history of failed crease operation, low eyelid crease height, thick skin, and slight ptosis. In clinical practice, it is not uncommon to come across young male patients who present after 3 failed operations for low eyelid crease. (Refer to the section on fixation types)

All eyelid creases become fainter for a certain amount of time. The mechanism behind the weakening of the crease is similar to that behind the formation of scar tissues. A scar widens if the tissue are approximated over a wide wound or if the scar is subjected movement (e.g. joint surface), and the eyelid crease is subjected to similar conditions. The postoperative eyelid crease becomes faint during the wound remodeling phase because the fixation becomes loose from several factors (hematoma, edema, tension, and blinking) prior to the adhesion finally setting in for the permanent crease. In this context, all operations that depend on sutures to withhold the tension across a wound must take into account the loosening of these sutures until the formation of adhesion. This is the same mechanism behind which ptosis correction is followed by a certain amount of eyelid margin descent. Severe ptosis requires relatively greater amount of advancement, which leads to greater tension across tissues and suture and subsequent postoperative descent of eyelid height (i.e. partial relapse of ptosis). This can be considered as a cheese-wiring effect of the suture through tissue.

Post-operative factors for faint eyelid crease

Operative factors that cause fading of the eyelid crease should be considered for the following situations.

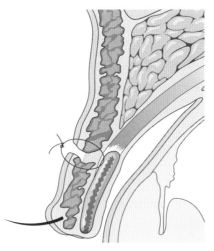

FIGURE 1-32 • A single fixation for tarsal fixation and skin closure.

This fixation should only be used as auxiliary sutures to reinforce permanent buried sutures or as guiding sutures to prevent the formation of multiple eyelid creases.

Skin-to-tarsal plate fixation without buried fixation (FIGURE 1-32)

A simple fixation that incorporates the skin closure and crease fixation to tarsal plate often results in faint crease. Buried fixations between orbicularis muscle and tarsal plate are much more secure. (The author uses this skin-to-tarsal fixation as an auxiliary method to augment the buried permanent sutures.)

Fixation of crease on the strength of fixation sutures alone without pretarsal soft tissue excision

This is a major problem in non-incisional eyelid crease operations with simple continuous fixations. Even though the suture material is permanent, the tension between the tissues eventually wins out the strength of fixation, which leads to loosening of the tissues. Ultimately, any fixation that ignores the need for tissue adhesion will fail over time, when subjected to repeated movement and prolonged tension.

Lower fixation

Lower fixation makes shallow fold or loss of fold.

Interposition of fat between anterior and posterior lamellae

Inadvertent interposition of the fat in this space prevents adhesion from forming between the layers. This is especially a common problem in the medial eyelid, where the excess of orbital fat can lead to fixation failure. If this is the case, the fat should be removed as a preventative measure against crease failure.

Inadequate number of buried fixation sutures

The number of buried fixation sutures should be higher in the presence of factors, which make crease faint.

Severe edema or hematoma

The change in tissue volume causes fixation sutures to become loose, which in turn causes the eyelid creases to fade or disappear.

Rubbing eyes

Patient who habitually rubs eyelids (e.g. atopic dermatitis) tend to have a difficult time keeping a postoperative eyelid crease.

Miscellaneous inappropriateness of fixation method

An example of this is strangulating sutures that cause focal tissue necrosis and fixation failure. Therefore, the first and the second sutures should be tied more loosely until the tension can be distributed more evenly across all fixation sutures.

CLASSIFICATION OF FIXATION TECHNIQUES

In the eyelid crease operation, a fixation is defined as a surgically created connection between the anterior lamella (the flap including the skin and the orbicularis oculi muscle) and the posterior lamella (tarsus, aponeurosis, and Müller's muscle).

Such a fixation can be considered in the following three characteristics.
- Location of fixation
- Tissues under fixation
- Direction of fixation

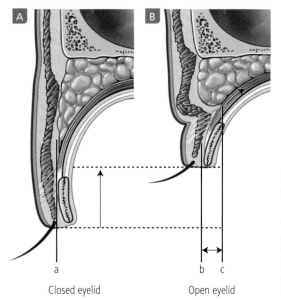

a
Closed eyelid

b c
Open eyelid

FIGURE 1-33 • High fixation causes posterior retraction of the eyelid crease, which creates a deep fold.

Principle: The levator palpebrae muscle moves the tarsal plate superiorly and posteriorly.

A. The lower border of tarsal plate of retracted eyelid (b) is at the same depth as the upper border of tarsal plate of closed eyelids (a). **B.** With the eyelid retracted, the location of the levator muscle with the fixation sutures are near 'c'. The distance between lines 'b' and 'c' is the depth of eyelid crease. Therefore the height of fixation point 'c' defines the fold depth.

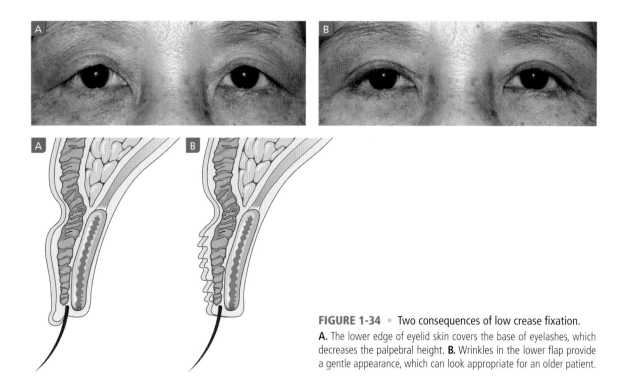

FIGURE 1-34 • Two consequences of low crease fixation.
A. The lower edge of eyelid skin covers the base of eyelashes, which decreases the palpebral height. **B.** Wrinkles in the lower flap provide a gentle appearance, which can look appropriate for an older patient.

Location of fixation

The average height of tarsal plate is 8.8mm in the Korean population. (Hwang) The fixation height on the tarsal plate can change the depth of eyelid crease. A high fixation will stretch the skin on the lower flap skin, which will create a deep fold with ectropion (**FIGURE 1-33**). In contrast, a low fixation creates a shallow crease with the lower flap skin covering the base of eyelashes. To create a crease of moderate depth, the lower flap should be fixated high enough on the tarsal plate such that the skin of the lower flap does not cover the roots of eyelashes. The eyelid should end with a slight ectropion, which becomes neutral over time.

In patients with thin and wrinkled skin and in elderly patients, the skin should not be fully extended. The height of fixation should be adjusted according to the factors influencing the eyelid resistance and the type of operation.

Lower fixation

Preoperative examination of the eyelids with a gentle touch of the stylus can yield important information on two potential variations of lower fixation (**FIGURE 1-34**).

Lax skin covering the palpebral fissure

In this variation, the lower edge of upper eyelid skin rests on top of the eyelashes and decreases the height of palpebral fissure. For female patients, this can create a difficulty in applying eyeliner along the lashes. To avoid this problem in patients who demonstrate such skin laxity, the crease should be fixated to a higher location (deeper fixation).

Slight wrinkling of the lower flap skin without sagging skin

If the wrinkling is not severe, the crease does not need to be fixated deeply to avoid creating unnaturally stretched eyelid skin. For elderly patients, slight wrinkling looks more natural and gentle than taut skin without any wrinkles.

When I perform these fixations, the upper of the tarsus is an excellent land mark. because the fixation points may be slightly moved based on the upper border of the tarsus to control the final results.

Height of fixation

Compared to the skin incision, the medial portion of crease is fixated at a higher

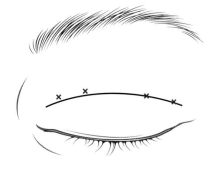

FIGURE 1-35 • Crease fixation vs. incision.
The height of crease fixation varies along the incision line. Medially, the crease is fixated higher than the incision line, whereas it is fixated at about a height equal to that of the incision line in the lateral portion of the eyelid. In the medial side, the author applies perform fixation at two points (upper border of tarsal plate and levator aponeurosis).

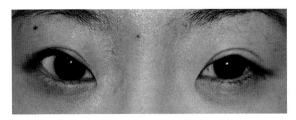

FIGURE 1-36 • The double fold line weakens at the medial side, and the upper eyelid hoods the palpebral fissure.

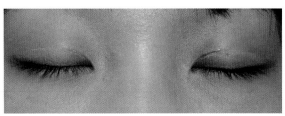

FIGURE 1-37 • As fixation is performed at higher levels at the medial side, depressed scars may form easily at the medial side.

location than the lateral crease **(FIGURE 1-35)**.

Reasons for higher fixation in the medial eyelid

1. Compared to the lateral side, the medial side has more pretarsal fat, more preaponeurotic fat, and more preMüller's muscle fat and fat infiltration in the Müller's muscle. These factors make it less likely for adhesions to form and contribute to decrease the height of eyelid crease. Much of this fat is difficult to excise because of the vascularity of the tissue. Also, fixation of the fat tissue can lead to cheese-wiring effect with adhesions forming subsequent to loosening of the fixation suture **(FIGURE 1-36, 1-37)**.

2. Another reason for high medial fixation is the elliptical fullness of the orbicularis oculi muscle is more pronounced in the medial portion of the eyelid, which can lead to hooding of the medial palpebral fissure. This situation requires an elliptical excision of the medial eyelid skin, along with low but upward fixation of the eyelid crease to create a distinct fold. High fixation of the crease to produce a distinct fold will create a depressed scar. 3. Also, the medial eyelid requires higher

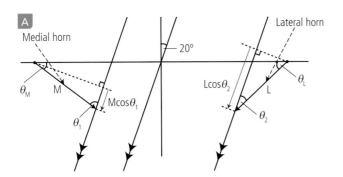 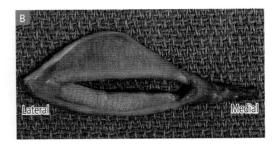

FIGURE 1-38 • The direction of fibers of the levator palpebrae muscle (Kakizaki).
A. As the medial horn is more horizontal than the lateral horn, the elevating power is weaker on the medial side compared to the lateral.
B. Upper border of tarsal plate is usually lower in medial side that lateral side.

fixation because the levator aponeurosis is more horizontal than the lateral horn. As such, the levator muscle has less of an influence on the medial portion of the eyelid margin **(FIGURE 1-38A)**. 4. High medial fixation is especially important for creating outside folds in the presence of epicanthal bands, to account for the increased resistance provided by the epicanthal fold. Should the medial portion of the eyelid crease become faint, patients will complain that the medial eyelid skin covering the eyelashes interferes with the make-up process. 5. Tarsus is usually smaller medially than laterally **(FIGURE 1-38B)**.

A fixation made above the upper tarsal border just to create a high crease can lead to depressed scar and ectropion. Prevention of these undesirable side effects requires advanced fixation techniques. This will be discussed more fully in a later section. 6. The bare area (i.e. aponeurosis is absent) on the medial side is larger than that of lateral side.

Tissues under fixation

Crease fixation is defined by a method of securing the tissues between the anterior (skin and orbicularis muscle) and posterior (tarsal plate, orbital septum, levator aponeurosis, and conjunctiva) lamellae.

Fixation of the anterior lamella

On the anterior lamella, the author fixates the orbicularis oculi muscle instead of dermis at the edge of lower eyelid flap. Dermotarsal fixation is a widely used terminology. However, electron microscopy of naturally occurring eyelid crease has demonstrated that the fibers from aponeurosis connect to the septa in the subcutaneous layer and connect indirectly to the skin through the orbicularis muscle. To simulate this, the author fixates the posterior lamella not to the dermis but to the oculi muscle. This fixation to the orbicularis muscle requires a big cuff of muscle to be available, which precludes excessive excision of the orbicularis muscle. Resection of orbicularis oculi muscle to improve adhesion should be avoided as it can lead to depressed scar.

Reasons for fixations to the orbicularis muscle

1. The dermis is very thin, but the orbicularis oculi muscle is thick. Fixations to the thicker tissue layer minimizes the chance of loosening or detaching of the fixed tissues.

2. The orbicularis oculi muscle is located more deeply than the dermis. Suture buried in the dermis can more easily result in inflammation and foreign body reactions around the sebaceous glands or sweat glands.

3. No gap is created between the inferior and superior flaps of orbicularis oculi muscles. When the dermis is fixed directly to the tarsus, a gap is created between the cut orbicularis oculi muscles, which may cause depressed scars even for non-incisional methods. This gap blocks the normal lymphatic and blood flow and may increase the duration of edema. The blood channels exist in discrete planes or tissue layers (e.g. dermal plexus, subdermal plexus, oculi muscle plexus), and a gap may cause blockage of the respective channels.

Fixation of the posterior lamella

The tarsal plate and levator aponeurosis are the major fixation tissues in the posterior lamella, though the septum may also be used. The following may be used as methods of fixation.

*   Exposed tarsus
*   Tarsus with attached aponeurosis
*   Directly to the aponeurosis superior to the tarsus
*   Dual fixation on the tarsus and the aponeurosis

- Anterior septum or posterior septum
- Direct fixation to the septum or aponeurosis in the lateral eyelid where the plate is absent.

A. Fixation to the exposed tarsus promotes adhesion between the anterior and posterior lamellae and is performed by exposing the tarsal plate of soft tissue. In this fixation, the force is applied exclusively to the tarsal plate, which is probably a weaker fixation than one that combines tarsal plate and aponeurosis. Also, removing all of the pretarsal tissue is traumatic. While this may promote better adhesion from scar formation, it may also diminish normal blood flow to the tissue as also be a cause for depressed scar.

B. Fixations to either the aponeurosis anterior to the tarsal plate or to the complex that includes the plate and the aponeurosis is much less traumatic and more secure, compared to fixation to an exposed tarsal plate.

C. Direct fixations can be made to the levator aponeurosis when the tarsal plate is particularly small (e.g. tarsal plate less than 6 mm). This method may be problematic in that ① there is a risk the fixation suture may irritate the conjunctival side. It may also cause ② ectropion, and may ③ limit the motion of the levator palpebrae muscle and cause fatigue eye. This method is not recommended.

D. The 3-point fixation method gathers the tarsal plate, the levator aponeurosis, and the lower flap with a single passage of the needle. This method slightly increases the amplitude of the levator aponeurosis (i.e. the degree of aponeurosis plication). Low tarsus and upper aponeurosis fixation has dual safety measures, which are prevention of ectropion and strengthening the weakness of the low fixation. The author prefers the partial thickness purchase of the tarsal plate with the needle for a variety of cases. The suture is passed through a partial thickness of tarsal plate, the aponeurosis above the tarsal plate, and then through the orbicularis oculi muscle. Because of the tissues involved, the author calls this method TAO (Tarsus, Aponeurosis, Orbicularis) fixation.

TAO Fixation

- Tarsal plate – The sutures are passed through a partial thickness of the plate. This portion of the fixation should not be too high to avoid stretching of the lower flap.

- Levator aponeurosis – The suture is then passed through the aponeurosis superior to the upper tarsal border.
- Orbicularis oculi muscle – The fixation is complete with a purchase of the orbicularis muscle near the dermis.

E. Fixation to the orbital septum

Some operators prefer fixation of the posterior lamella using the anterior or posterior septum, instead of the tarsal plate or the levator aponeurosis. This method can be appropriate in special circumstances. The posterior septum is a type of an aponeurotic sheath, and fixation to this tissue is, though slightly weak, not too different from fixation to the aponeurosis itself. The downside to using the posterior septum is that it can be sensitive to weakening or deepening of the eyelid crease. The anterior septum near the levator aponeurosis can be made into a turn-over flap, fixation to which decreases the risk of depressed scars.

In conclusion, the methods described in A and C are not recommended. Methods B, D, and E are useful.

Crease fixation in the lateral eyelid in the elderly

In the lateral eyelid, the tarsal plate is absent. In younger patients, the surgically created eyelid crease continues laterally without any fixations in this region, but this is usually not the case in the elderly. The absence of tarsal plate in the lateral eye requires that the crease fixation be performed on the aponeurosis or the septum **(FIGURE 1-40)**. However, the aponeurosis insert to the Whitnall's tubercle which is deep inside of the orbital rim. Therefore direct fixation to this point of the aponeurosis may create a deep and abruptly ending crease line. This should be avoided. Instead, long thread suture fixation or lateral extension of aponeurosis is appropriate site to which the fixation is performed **(FIGURE 1-39)**. (Detailed discussion in Aging Blepharoplasty, Chapter 2.)

Dynamic fold

Generally, a satisfactory upper eyelid crease can be characterized as having the desired length, curvatures, and depth with a minimal incisional scar. Here, the

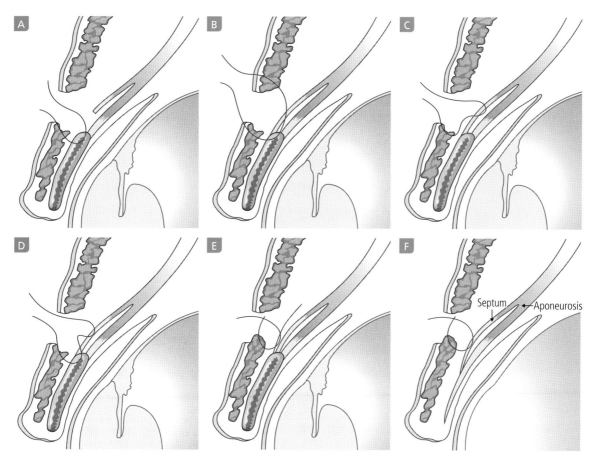

FIGURE 1-39 • Various fixation methods for the posterior lamella.
A. Removal of the pretarsal soft tissue and fixation to the exposed tarsal plate
B. Concomitant fixation to the pretarsal levator aponeurosis and tarsal plate
C. Direct fixation to the upper levator aponeurosis
D. Concomitant fixation to the tarsal plate and the levator aponeurosis in separate bites (TAO fixation)
E. Fixation to the septum in the lateral portion of eyelid
F. Fixation to the septum or aponeurosis in the lateral portion of eyelid

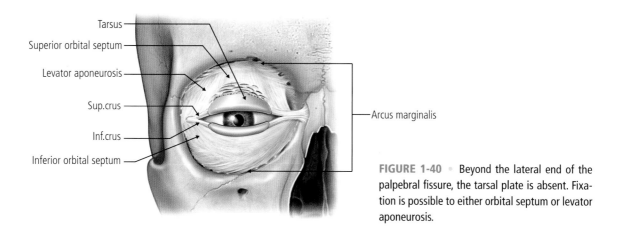

FIGURE 1-40 • Beyond the lateral end of the palpebral fissure, the tarsal plate is absent. Fixation is possible to either orbital septum or levator aponeurosis.

author would like to discuss a more advanced form of eyelid crease. In addition to the standard criteria mentioned above, the ideal eyelid crease should not contain a scar, which becomes noticeable with closing of eyelids or with downgaze. The crease should be inconspicuous on closed eyelids and should begin to show as a gentle crease or fold with opening of the lids, which is the definition of a dynamic fold. On closed eyelids, the depressed scar and the supratarsal fold may appear similar but should be differentiated. Of the two, depressed scar is to be avoided, whereas a natural crease is welcomed. This depends on the type of fixation used.

The fixation is performed on the orbicularis oculi muscle without incorporating the dermis.

1. TAO fixation is performed.

- The fixation is performed on the orbicularis oculi muscle without incorporating the dermis.

- The needle is passed through a partial thickness of tarsal plate, at a level similar to or slightly higher than the desired crease height. Too high of a fixation can stretch the lower flap and can also lead to depressed scar and ectropion with closed eyelids.

- The aponeurosis superior to the upper tarsal border should be stretched and fixed without much tension. This added tension from the aponeurosis helps to prevent the crease from fading. The rationale for the partial thickness bite of tarsal plate is to prevent stretching of the lower flap from this tension of levator aponeurosis (FIGURE 1-41).

- The needle is passed through the orbicularis oculi muscle near the skin. Purchasing a bite of the orbicularis muscle far away from the skin can lead to inconsistencies in the crease height. However, superficial fixation should also be avoided, as it can lead to slight dimpling of the skin (FIGURE 1-42).

2. Once the needle has passed through all three layers, the suture ends are gently tied. Because the fixation is not too high on the tarsal plate or the aponeurosis, the resulting crease appears more natural. This fixation avoids the ectropion and depressed scars associated with downgaze. At the same time, the fixation decreases the likelihood of loosening by incorporating the aponeurosis into the fixation.

This method is especially important for non-incision and partial incision

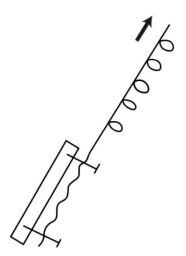

FIGURE 1-41 ◦ A mechanical schematic of a plank and elastic fiber.
Despite the tension from the upper end, the nail prevents stretching of the lower portion of the fiber. The partial thickness bite of the tarsal plate serves as the nail that prevents transmission of tension from the levator to the lower flap.

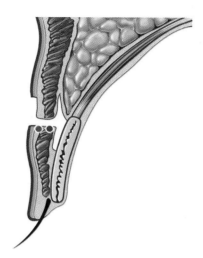

FIGURE 1-42 ◦ Fixation of the orbicularis muscle.
The needle is passed through the orbicularis oculi muscle near the skin (blue dot). Deep fixation (red dot) decreases the consistency of crease height and depth. The fixation to the orbicularis muscle should be made between these two depths.

operations because partial depressions are more conspicuous than depression of the whole incisional scar.

In younger patients, the author uses 4 TAO fixations per eyelid. The two medial fixations are performed at the level of the desired eyelid crease. The remaining two lateral sutures are fixated 1 mm higher than the crease **(FIGURE 1-43)**.

Mechanism of TAO fixation

1. The tarsal fixation prevents stretching of the lower skin flap
2. Fixation to the levator above the tarsal border
3. Orbicularis muscle fixation

Advantages of TAO fixation

1. This method avoids the creation of ectropic, deep crease. It also decreases the likelihood of the crease loosening.
2. The recovery is quick. Because the fixation is not too high on tarsal plate, the conversion from deep fold to shallow crease takes less time.
3. Partial incision method can create the formation of delayed fold.
4. The operation does not decrease the levator function. (Refer to the section on eyelid

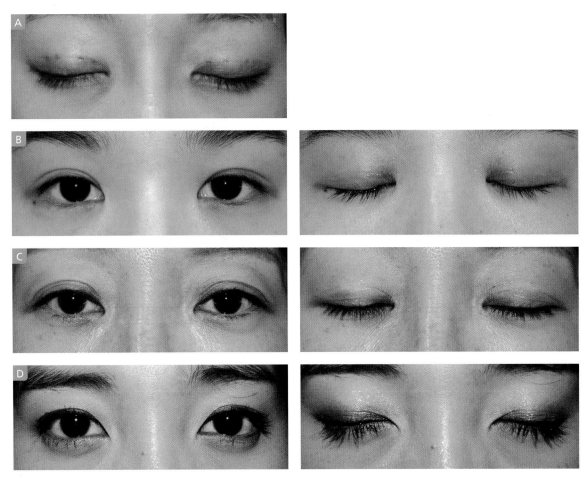

FIGURE 1-43 • **A.** Depressed scars are noticeable even for non-incisional methods. **B.** Advanced eyelid creases are inconspicuous on closed eyelids. It does not have any depressions, and becomes noticeable only when the eyelids are open. **C.** These are surgically created eyelid creases. **D.** Natural eyelid creases.
No differences are noted in the eyelid creases between Patients **C** and **D**.

height, p-4)

5. The technique is applicable in a variety of situations.

Miscellaneous

Appropriate uses for TAO fixation

1. Fixation of medial eyelid creases: The fixation can easily come undone in the medial side because of the difference in the height of tarsal plate. On the other hand, a high fixation directly to the aponeurosis without tarsal plate may lead to

WAIT A MINUTE!

DYNAMIC VERSUS STATIC EYELID CREASE

The topic of dynamic versus static crease has been discussed with some confusion. One school of thought is "dynamic eyelid crease is inconspicuous in closed eyelids, whereas the static creases are visible." Another group of operators describes dynamic crease to be a result of fixation to the levator aponeurosis or septum (dynamic) as opposed to tarsal plate (static). The author believes this to be a problem of terminology.

The aponeurosis, tarsal plate, and septum do not possess innate elasticity. Even if the aponeurosis is considered to be more dynamic than the tarsal plate because it contracts with the Müller's muscle, all eyelid creases can be dynamic creases

Non-dynamic creases can be found in ptosis patients. In these patients, the levator muscle is not as elastic, and the crease does not change much regardless of the gaze. The crease in patients with ptosis is static. Therefore, the creation of advanced eyelid crease is possible regardless of the tissue that is used for fixation, as long as the proper techniques are employed.

depression and conspicuousness of eyelid crease with downward gaze.

2. If the tarsal plate is small, the tarsal fixation may not adequately support the lower flap. Direct fixation to the aponeurosis to alleviate this problem will result in the 'lazy eye' appearance.

3. Patient requests low eyelid creases (inside fold). High fixation can lead to ectropion, but low fixation may not be secure. TAO fixation will address both of these concerns.

4. Pre-existing ectropion from previous operation. In such patients, ectropion can recur easily, yet methods that avoid ectropion often produce creases that tend to fade or disappear. TAO fixation addresses the ectropion by the low fixation to the tarsal plate. However, the fixation to aponeurosis prevents the disappearance of eyelid crease.

5. In ptosis correction, the crease is secure in the medial and central portion of the eyelid. However, it tends to fade in the lateral portion of eyelid, where the levator was not advanced. In such cases, TAO fixation can simulate the levator advancement in the lateral point because of the fixation of levator muscle.. The crease tends to be secure because the fixation has a plication effect on the aponeurosis.

6. With skin shortage resulting from prior operation, even a lower fixation may result in ectropion because of the out-stretched lower flap skin. In such cases,

the lower flap is secured relatively low on the tarsal plate to minimize the tension from above, with a levator aponeurosis fixation as per usual TAO fixation. The lower flap skin should remain relatively tension free even after closure **(FIGURE 1-41)**.

7. In patients with weak levator function, eyelid crease operation can result in descent of the upper eyelid margin. (Refer to section on palpebral height, p-3) TAO fixation has a slight plication effect on the levator muscle and can alleviate some decrease in fissure height.

Direction of fixation

Fixations are performed in a radial direction. Medially, the orbicularis muscle should be fixed to the tarsal plate at a location more medial to the orbicularis muscle. Laterally, the orbicularis oculi muscle is fixed to a posterior element (tarsal plate, aponeurosis, or septum) at a more lateral location. The anterior surface of globe is not a flat surface, and the eyelid does not move straight up and down. The levator palpebrae aponeurosis spreads in a fan shape. When the muscle contracts, the aponeurosis gathers towards the center, which implies that the fixations in the medial and lateral eyelid should compensate for this horizontal translation. During the operation, fixating the tarsal plate first will lead to fixation of the flaps in a more central direction.

In other words, the medial fixation should be performed such that the needle is first passed through the tarsal plate and then passed through the orbicularis muscle

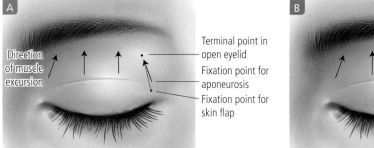
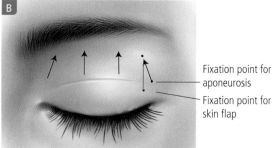

FIGURE 1-44 • Fixation points between lower flap and tarsal plate in relation to eyelid movement. (Red arrows represent movement of lower flap with eyelid retraction.)

A. A strictly vertical relationship between fixation points will result in the lower flap being retracted toward a medial point, which is undesirable.

B. A proper fixation of the lower skin flap should compensate horizontally and should result in the skin flap being raised vertically.

at a more lateral location. Conversely, lateral fixation should incorporate tarsal plate first and then the orbicularis muscle at a more medial location **(FIGURE 1-44 & 1-45)**.

Length of eyelid creases

In attractive eyelids, supratarsal creases begin 2-3 mm away from the medial canthus and extend 4-6 mm beyond the lateral canthus. The crease can be shorter in introverted persons and in male patients. When excising the skin, the incision line should deflect upwards at a point 4-6 mm is the turning point beyond the lateral canthus. (Refer to **FIGURE 1-46**.)

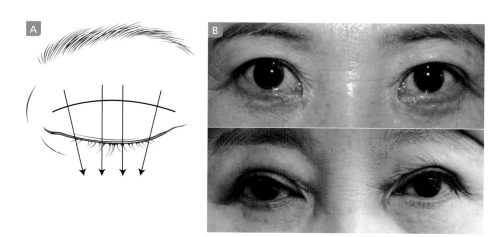

FIGURE 1-45 • **A.** Direction of fixation. The fixations should go from the tarsal plate medially to the orbicularis muscle to compensate for the radial movement of the aponeurosis. In the center portion of the eyelid, it is performed vertically. The outward fixation is needed for the medial and lateral, with medial fixation requiring more compensation. **B.** The lack of medial compensation can result in the wrinkles observed superior to the double fold.

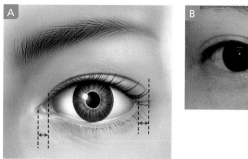
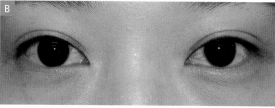

FIGURE 1-46 • Length of eyelid creases.
Ideally, the crease begins 2-3 mm from the medial canthus and extends 4-6 mm past the lateral canthus.

KNOT TYING

The author ties the fixation sutures using 4-6 knots for the PDS suture. Three knots are can often leads to undoing of the suture tie. The PDS maintains its strength for 6 months, after which it undergoes absorption. The fixation sutures are tied with the first and second knots being made fairly loose to prevent necrosis of tissue within the suture loop. The remaining two knots should be tied strongly to prevent the knot from becoming undone.

Nylon suture material may be used. Many surgeons probably have experienced sustained double folds after removal of the nylon suture due to inflammation even at 2 months after operation. PDS maintains power for at least 2 months.

SKIN SUTURE

As with other surgical procedures, the edges of skin incision should be approximated and closed in an everted manner. To avoid a gap in the orbicularis muscles between the upper and lower flaps, the skin sutures should incorporate the orbicularis muscle. For incisional operations, few intermittent sutures are placed to secure the skin and orbicularis muscle to the tarsal plate. These sutures offload the tension from buried fixation sutures **(FIGURE 1-47)** and also help to create adhesion. The remainder of skin may be closed using a continuous running suture.

In elderly patients, the lateral portion of the incision where is no fold should be closed with vertical mattress sutures to ensure proper eversion of the wound margins.

The suture should be done finely. If the lower skin flap is connected to the levator complex via buried fixation suture, the likelihood of skin dislocation is high **(FIGURE 1-48)**. To prevent this, the skin sutures should be spaced closely. Interlocking sutures are preferred over simple continuous sutures because the later method can result in zig-zag shape of the incision line.

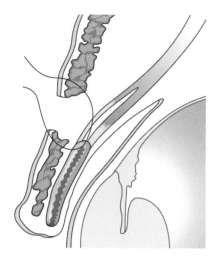

FIGURE 1-47 • At times, skin closing sutures can incorporate the orbicularis muscle and the tarsal plate.

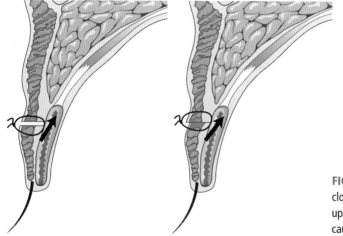

FIGURE 1-48 • If the skin sutures are not spaced closely, the buried fixation sutures may translate the upward tension to the inferior skin flap, which will cause dislocation of the wound margin.

In the elderly, excision of redundant skin can lead to a large difference in the skin thickness between the upper and lower flaps. In such cases, the operator should compensate for the difference by purchasing a partial thickness bite of the upper flap skin and a full thickness bite of the lower flap skin.

FREQUENTLY ASKED QUESTIONS

Q **HOW SHOULD EYELID CREASE OPERATION BE PERFORMED IN A PATIENT WITH ASYMMETRIC EYE SIZES?**

A The operator must evaluate the cause of this asymmetry and employ the method that is appropriate for that cause. The following examples represent more common causes of such asymmetry.

1. The asymmetry results from unilateral ptosis (FIGURE 1-49).

This represents a difference in the function of the levator muscle between the two eyelids. In such patients, correction of the ptotic eyelid should be recommended prior to the eyelid crease operation. If the unilateral ptosis is extremely mild or if the patient does not wish for a ptosis operation, then the eyelid crease should be designed at a lower height in the ptotic ("smaller") eyelid and at a relatively higher position in the non-ptotic ("larger") eye. In this case, the patient should be informed in advance that the eyelid creases will look asymmetric with downgaze or with closing of eyelids.

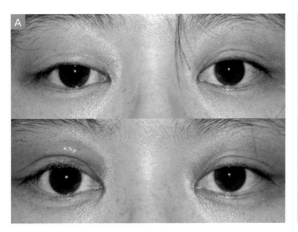 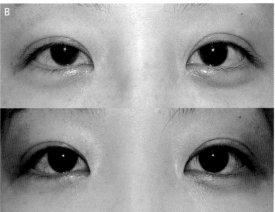

FIGURE 1-49 • The ptosis in the right eyelid was addressed with levator advancement.

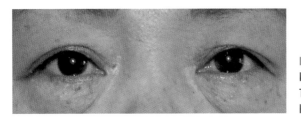

FIGURE 1-50 • The eyelid crease appears to be lower on the left eyelid because the skin laxity is greater in the left eyelid. To achieve symmetry, the skin excision should be greater in the left eyelid.

2. The asymmetry is in dermatochalasis (FIGURE 1-50).

The eyelid crease is set at the same height between both upper eyelids. The skin excision should be greater in the eyelid with greater skin sagging. Asymmetry of skin laxity should not be addressed by differing the height of the crease alone. Not only is that approach technically challenging, and even successful attempt will result in asymmetry of the eyelid crease with downgaze and upgaze (FIGURE 1-50). The differential excision of eyelid skin is discussed in Chapter 2.

3. The asymmetry is in the eyebrow position (FIGURE 1-51).

The proper approach is to obtain symmetry of the eyebrows (i.e. brow lift) prior to eyelid crease operation. If the operation is too inconvenient or if the patient does not wish for it, a greater amount of skin should be excised on the side with the lower eyebrow.

4. The asymmetry is in the shape of eyelid crease itself (FIGURE 1-52).

Asymmetry in the shape or height of the eyelid crease is relatively conspicuous. An exception can be made for asymmetry of inside folds, which can be mistaken for unilateral ptosis. An eyelid with an extremely low crease or without a crease

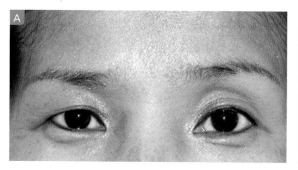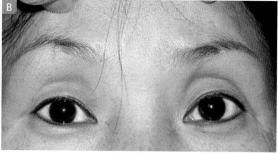

FIGURE 1-51 • **A.** The right eye appears to be smaller (suggesting unilateral ptosis of right eyelid). **B.** Manual elevation of both brows reveals the absence of true ptosis on the right eyelid. The asymmetry is caused by the hollowness in the left eyelid and the asymmetry of the eyebrows.

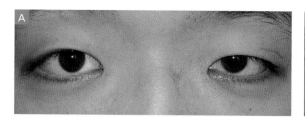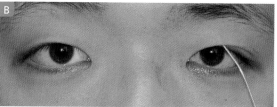

FIGURE 1-52 • **A.** The inside fold is higher on the right side, which makes the right eye appear to be larger than the left eye. In this case, the eyelid crease operation should be performed the same way for both eyelids. **B.** Simulation of the eyelid crease on the left side demonstrates the underlying symmetry in the palpebral fissure.

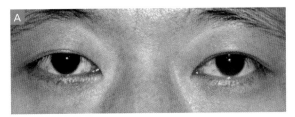 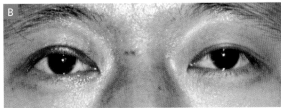

FIGURE 1-53 • **A.** The right eye appears to be smaller because the crease is faint on that side. **B.** After eyelid crease operation, the eyes appear to be more symmetric.

at all has more skin laxity, which tends to make the eyelid appear lower than it really it. In such cases, the eyelid crease operation should proceed as usual with the eyelid creases set at the same height.

The main problem in addressing asymmetric eyelids by etiology is the very challenge in recognizing the cause in the first place.

Methods for discriminating the cause of asymmetry

- Both eyelids are elevated just so the eyelid skin no longer rests on the base of eyelashes. If the upper eyelid margins are asymmetric, then the cause is asymmetry in levator function (i.e. unilateral ptosis).
- Upon simulating eyelid crease with stylus in both eyelids, the remaining asymmetry is due to a difference in the levator function.
- In downgaze, skin laxity no longer becomes a cause for asymmetry. Another method of evaluating dermatochalasis as a cause of asymmetry is to have the patient lay supine. However, this method is not as accurate and should be used as an adjunctive examination.

5. Asymmetry is due to difference in the eyelid crease.
The eye with faint eyelid crease tends to appear smaller (**FIGURE 1-53**).

6. Asymmetry is due to the lower eyelid height.
All other factors being equal, asymmetry in palpebral fissure height can be attributed to the difference in the height of the lower eyelid margin.

Q SHOULD SKIN EXCISION BE PERFORMED IN YOUNG PATIENTS WITH MINOR LAXITY?

A In the sitting position, the eyelid creases should be simulated with a stylus. The eyelids should be examined with and

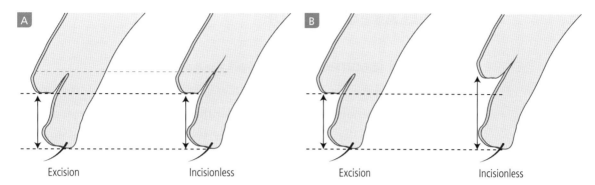

| A | Excision | Incisionless | B | Excision | Incisionless |

FIGURE 1-54 • **A.** On primary gaze, the height of double fold is the same between incision and non-incision operations. **B.** On downgaze, the double fold is taller for the non-incision method, which can easily lead to pretarsal bulkiness.

without the elevation of the eyebrows by an assistant. The assistant should elevate the eyebrow such that the eyelid skin is stretched 80-90% of the full length. If the examination reveals severe drooping of the skin above the eyelid crease, skin excision is recommended. Skin excision is not needed unless the need can be clearly demonstrated by the examination.

Usually, skin excision is appropriate only if the laxity is greater than 3 mm. For minor skin laxity, the skin excision does not provide enough benefit in exchanged for the increased risk of scarring. Exceptions can be made for extremely bulky eyelids for which orbital fat excision is inadequate for debulking. In such cases, excisions of eyelid skin may be helpful, even if the amount of skin excision ends up being less than 3 mm in width.

Pretarsal bulkiness is another major issue that can easily be overlooked. If the height of the eyelid crease is the same between the non-incision and the incision operation, the pretarsal volume will also be the same on primary gaze. However, all of this changes with downgaze, by which the pretarsal bulk will appear greater for non-incision method. If this is expected, it is better to set the eyelid crease low and excise the skin because pretarsal bulkiness is more common with the non-incision method **(FIGURE 1-54)**.

KEYPOINT 🔒

Without skin excision, the crease should be designed at a higher position than the one designed with skin excision. The following observations apply to excision-less operation.

- The recovery period is longer.
- Pretarsal bulkiness is a potential issue, especially with downgaze.
- Higher eyelid creases are prone to become deeper folds.

Considerations for low crease operations with skin excision.

- Skin laxity may develop sooner than later.
- Incisional scar will be more noticeable.

MISCELLANEOUS ISSUE

Prolapse of lacrimal gland (FIGURE 1-55 & 1-56)

The lacrimal gland is easily confused with lateral fat bulging. However, the bulging location is more inferior for the gland than for the fat tissue. The lacrimal gland is much firmer than fat tissue and is paler in color. With prolapse or inferior displacement, the lacrimal gland should be dissected and sutured to the internal periosteum of the upper orbital rim, to relocate it into the lacrimal gland fossa and to prevent relapse. The gland should be separated and freed from surrounding tissue before suturing to the periosteum. Because the prolapse can easily recur, the gland should be securely fixated in the destination with multiple sutures.

When performing partial excision, the gland should be tied and excised to prevent a lacrimal fistula from forming. If a fistula occurs from laceration of the lacrimal ductules, the cut ductile is tied or cauterized. A drain is inserted in that position and left in place. When the amount of lacrimal discharge is significantly decreased, the drain can be removed.

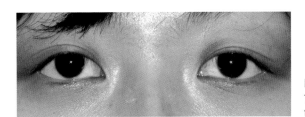

FIGURE 1-55 • A case of lacrimal gland prolapse.
The lacrimal gland prolapse is usually located lower than bulging position of lateral orbital fat.

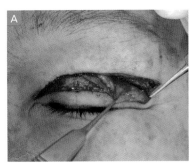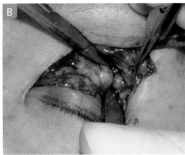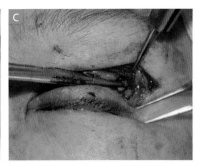

FIGURE 1-56 • Relocation of the lacrimal gland.
A. Prolapsed lacrimal gland. **B.** The lacrimal gland is dissected from surrounding tissue. A subperiosteal space is dissected at the orbital rim.
C. The lacrimal gland is buried in this space, and the periosteum is closed.

📑 REFERENCES

1. Flower RS : Upper blepharoplasty by eyelid invagination; Anchor blepharoplasty. Clin Plast Surg 20(2):193-207, 1993.
2. Fagien S : Temporary management of upper lid ptosis, lid malposition and eyelid fissure asymmetry with botulinum toxin type A) Plast Reconstr Surg 114:1892, 2004.
3. Ahn HB, Lee YI : The study of anatomic relationship between the Müller muscle and tarsus in Asian upper eyelid. Ophthl Plast Reconstr Surg 26(50):334-338, 2010.
4. Morikawa K, Yamamoto H : Scanning electron microscopic study on double and single eyelids in orientals. Aesth Plast Surg 25:20-24, 2001.

02

UPPER BLEPHAROPLASTY FOR THE ELDERLY

- Preoperative planning
- Operative details
- Ancillary procedures
- Miscellaneous issues
- Infrabrow blepharoplasty
- Things to keep in mind after upper eyelid surgery

PREOPERATIVE PLANNING

In elderly patients, the objective of blepharoplasty is not to simply create attractive eyelids but to create eyelids that appear youthful but are harmonious with rest of the visage. Correction of droopy upper eyelid skin is the most important goal of blepharoplasty in elderly patients. This goal can be accomplished with or without the creation of an eyelid crease, according to patient preference. However, the author tends to recommend in favor of the eyelid crease because it helps to prevent or delay the recurrence of dermatochalasis. If the patient does not wish for an eyelid crease, a compromise can be made for a low inconspicuous crease. It is important to note that a high percentage of East Asian men prefer not to have eyelid creases for social reasons. Elevated eyebrows are common in elderly patients, who have been compensating for the dermatochalasis with the forehead muscle. In such patients, the blepharoplasty should be performed with the postoperative descent of eyebrows in mind.

Elderly patients tend to have relatively thin upper eyelid skin, thin orbicularis oculi muscle, and little retro-orbicularis fat. In most cases, skin excision alone is sufficient without removal of deeper connective tissues. Also, excessive excision of connective tissue tends to prolong recovery period in elderly patients. In contrast to younger patients, outstretching of the pretarsal skin can lead to a highly unnatural look in elderly patients. To avoid this, the lower skin flap must be fixed while allowing for laxity.

OPERATIVE DETAILS

Incision design

The skin excision requires two incision lines. The bottom line defines the contour of the new eyelid crease, whereas the top line defines the width of skin excision.

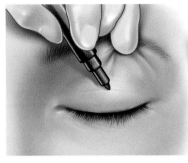 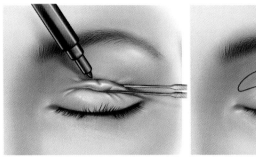 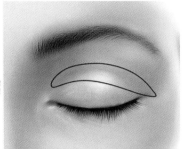

FIGURE 2-1 • In conventional method of design, the crease is designed to be 7-9 mm above the central eyelash line of the upper eyelid.

FIGURE 2-2 • The amount of skin excision is evaluated using a forceps. The upper eyelid skin is pinched to the extent that the eyelashes are everted. The upper incision line is drawn at the height defined by the forceps pinch.

Method I) Conventional blepharoplasty

Designing the crease shape (inferior incision line) (FIGURE 2-1, 2-2)

The inferior incision line is usually designed 7-9 mm superior to the eyelash line. Another method is to design a line along the supratarsal border, by everting the eyelid and measuring the height of tarsal plate. (e.g. Flower's method)

Deciding the amount of skin excision (superior incision line)

Using a forceps, the eyelid skin is pinched to identify the amount of skin excision excision needed to evert the eyelashes.

Method II) The author's method

Designing the crease shape (inferior incision line)

With the patient in sitting position, an assistant manually elevates the patient's eyebrows such that the upper eyelid skin is stretched to 80-90% of the length of fully stretched upper eyelid skin. The operator uses a stylus to simulate a variety of eyelid crease shapes, while the patient views herself in the mirror. Upon a thorough discussion with the patient, the operator confirms the most desirable shape of eyelid crease. If this evaluation process is performed with the eyelid skin fully stretched, the eyelid crease will appear very unnatural.

Elderly patients with pre-existing supratarsal crease

Whether to preserve the existing fold or to modify the fold shape is discussed with the patient in the same manner as described above (with the skin stretched 80-90% of full length). In addition, the preoperative discussion should include whether the patient would like to have the new eyelid crease to be higher, lower, or in a different shape, compared to that of the pre-existing crease.

Deciding the amount of skin excision (superior incision line)

This part of the examination continues with the eyebrows elevated, as described above. Once the inferior incision line has been designed, the operator should measure the distance between the lower lid margin to the inferior line, using a caliper, along the midpupillary line. The eyebrow is then allowed to descend into the natural height, which would bring down the height of lower incision line. The caliper from previous measurement is used to mark a position above the lower incision line, which marks the central point of the upper incision line (FIGURE 2-3). This process of measuring and marking the upper incisional point is repeated two more times, vertically above the medial limbus and the lateral canthus. These three points are then used to draw out the upper incision line (FIGURE 2-4, 2-5).

In elderly patients, the skin and orbicularis oculi muscle represents the majority of soft tissue redundancy in the upper eyelid. Correction of this drooping soft

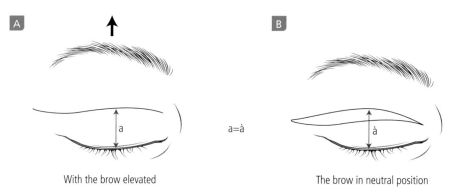

With the brow elevated	The brow in neutral position

FIGURE 2-3 • Determination of the incision line.
A. With the brow elevated as described in the main text, the lower incision is designed using an eyelid stylus. A caliper is used to measure the height of this crease at the midpupillary line (distance 'a'). **B.** With the eyebrow in its neutral state, the measuring caliper is used to mark the same height at the midpupillary line. Because of the descent of eyebrow and the upper eyelid skin, the caliper will now indicate a new point on the eyelid that represents the prior height of lower incision line. (Distance 'a' = Distance 'à').

tissue requires excision of both skin and orbicularis muscle. A large skin excision can cause brow ptosis, however. To avoid this problem, a more moderate amount of skin can be excised, while excising a portion of the orbicularis muscle and underlying connective tissue. This combined approach to excision provides similar operative outcomes while minimizing the risk of brow ptosis. The only caveat to this approach is that the excision of orbicularis muscle in the upper flap should be avoided because it can lead to the formation of an additional crease (AKA "triple fold" in East Asian blepharoplasty vernacular). (**FIGURE 2-9**, Refer also to the section on multiple creases on p-125.)

The skin and orbicularis oculi muscle functions as a single unit in the upper eyelid. As such, both of the tissues age in unison (i.e. stretching, attenuation, atrophy, and drooping).

Few comments
- Excessive skin excision leads to drooping appearance of lateral area of eyelid skin. This aggravates crow's feet.
- Excision of soft tissue in the upper flap must be conservative, as overzealous excision of this area can result in triple fold.
- In hollow eyelids, the excision should be limited to the skin only, while preserving the orbicularis muscle and other connective tissues. The author avoids resection of orbicularis muscle in more than half of the elderly patients undergoing blepharoplasty. When muscle resection is unavoidable, the amount of resected muscle is always less than the amount of excised skin.

The author has experienced a disappointing outcome in a specific type of cases, in which the skin excision appeared to be adequate at the conclusion of the operation. In these cases, the eyebrows descended in the postoperative phase with return of skin drooping above the eyelid crease. To prevent this, the patient must be in a relaxed state of mind during the intraoperative examination, such that the eyebrows are allowed to fully descend. Then, the amount of skin excision is determined by designing the superior incision line, while an assistant gently depresses the eyebrows.

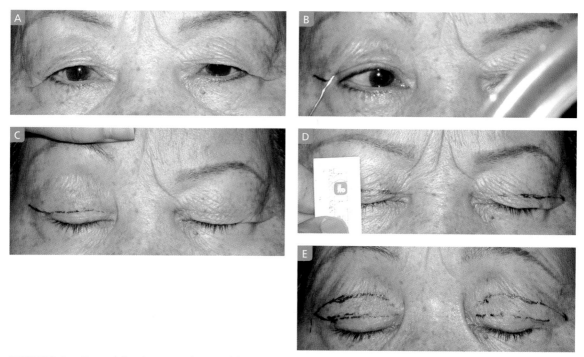

FIGURE 2-4 • Determining the crease shape and the amount of skin excision in elderly patients.
A. This elderly patient demonstrates significant dermatochalasis in the preoperative setting. **B.** With the upper eyelid skin stretched to 80-90% of its full length, the eyelid stylus is used to simulate various crease shapes until the desired crease is identified through discussion. **C.** With the eyebrow still elevated, the examiner measures the distance between the eyelid margin and the lower incision line. This patient wished for a crease 8 mm above the eyelid margin. **D.** To determine upper incision line, the eyebrow is allowed to return to the neutral position, which has resulted in the lower incision line being hidden below the drooping skin. The superior incision line is designed 8 mm above the eyelid margin. **E.** The eyebrow is elevated again to demonstrate the resulting incision lines, which outline the amount of skin to be excised.

Differential excision of eyelid skin

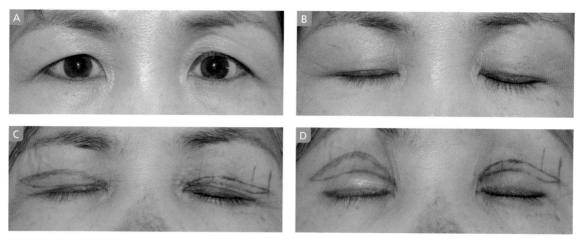

FIGURE 2-5 • **A & B.** Preoperative photographs. **C.** With closed eyes, inferior incision line appears asymmetric, while the superior incision line appears similar. The superior incision line is about 10 mm above the eyelid margin. **D.** When the eyebrows are elevated, the inferior incision lines appear symmetric. The superior incision line is higher in the right eyelid, which indicates greater amount of skin redundancy on the right side. Here, the inferior incision line is about 10 mm above the eyelid margin.

Length of incision

Medially, the incision is limited to the eyelid skin and should not invade into the nasal skin. Laterally, the incision should not extend more than 2 cm beyond the orbital rim. The skin is thicker outside of the eyelid region, and extending the incision outside of the eyelid increases the risk of scarring. For excessive skin redundancy, too large of a skin excision can lead to brow ptosis. In this case, the amount of excised skin should be reduced, while increasing the amount of excised orbicularis muscle. Because the skin and orbicularis muscle forms single unit, the amount of excision can be distributed from skin to the muscle. However, one must be careful not to allow the muscle excision to become a cause for triple fold.

Shape of incision

Consideration for the medial eyelid incision

The medial eyelid skin tends to have mild skin drooping, and dermatochalasis and brow ptosis are more severe in the lateral eyelid. The incision should change according to the degree of skin redundancy in the medial eyelid.

- Mild skin redundancy should result in a narrow width of skin excision design in the medial eyelid. As such, there is little length difference between the superior and inferior incisions **(FIGURE 2-6A)**.
- Moderate skin redundancy requires an incision design with considerable difference between the upper and lower incisions such that the incisions are medially extended **(FIGURE 2-6B)**.
- Severe skin redundancy can be accompanied by dermatochalasis on the nasal skin immediately adjacent to the eyelid border. In such cases, a back-cut is designed to prevent dog ear formation from the difference in skin length **(FIGURE 2-6C)**. The width of back-cut should not be wide because a wide back-cut can lead to band formation or hypertrophic scarring from excessive tension. And diluted Triamsinole solution is injected on the back-cut area to prevent from hypertropic scar formation.

Consideration for the lateral eyelid incision

The incision should follow the shape of the intended crease line and is upturned posterolaterally at a point where the crease should end. This inflection point is usually 4-6 mm past the lateral canthus. This inflection can be made a bit medial for patients who wish for shorter eyelid creases (**FIGURE 2-7, 2-8**).

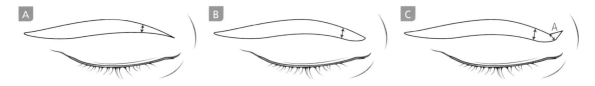

FIGURE 2-6 • The design of medial eyelid incision varies according to the amount of skin to be excised.
A. Minor skin redundancy requires minimal skin excision. **B.** Moderate skin redundancy requires medial extension of the excision. **C.** Severe skin redundancy requires a back-cut to address the difference in length between upper and lower incisions. The base of the back-cut triangle 'A' should be narrow, or a wide back-cut base will result in a band that appears similar to epicanthal fold.

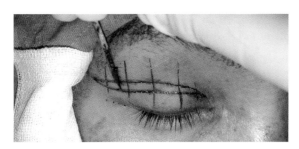

FIGURE 2-7 • The inflection point should be 4-6 mm beyond the lateral canthus (indicated by the ink stylus). A more laterally extended inflection point will turn the lateral portion of eyelid crease into one limb of the crow's feet. A shorter crease will not help in preventing the skin from drooping.

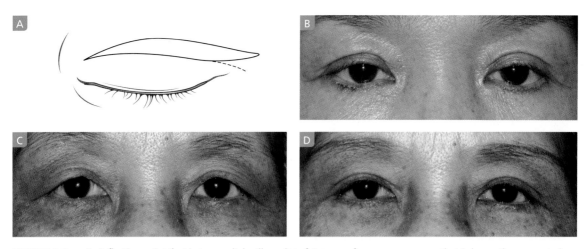

FIGURE 2-8 • An inflection point that is too medial will result in faintness of crease or a crease that is lower than expected. **A & B.** Creases that downturn in the lateral eyelid. **C.** Short creases that do not extend laterally. **D.** These eyelids look natural because the creases are at an even height through the full length of the eyelids.

Resection of orbicularis oculi muscle

In eyelids of average thickness, the orbicularis muscle should be resected along with skin excision. A cuff of 1-2 mm orbicularis muscle should be preserved next to the superior and inferior skin margins. The superior cuff prevents triple folds, and the inferior cuff prevents depressed scars **(FIGURE 2-9)**.

In thinner eyelids, however, the excision of soft tissue should be limited to the skin itself, while preserving the orbicularis oculi to avoid further hollowness of the eyelid. In the elderly, the eyelid is usually thin from skin redundancy and orbicularis oculi muscle atrophy. In this case, the lower flap should not be dissected, and the orbicularis muscle should not be excised. Violation of the lower flap integrity in the elderly eyelids can result in adhesion and stiffness of the pretarsal area and can also be followed by pigmentation or telangiectasia.

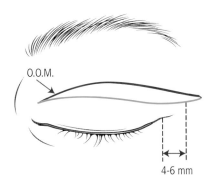

FIGURE 2-9 • A 1-2 mm cuff of orbicularis muscle cuff should be preserved both at the upper and lower excision margins. Excision of orbicularis oculi in the red area increases the risk of triple fold, and excision in the blue area increases the risk for depressed scar.

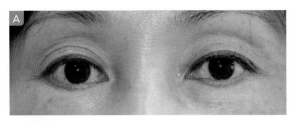

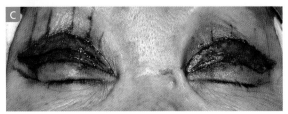

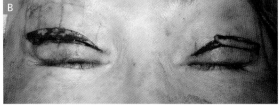

FIGURE 2-10 • In sunken eyelids with thin wrinkled skin, only the redundant portion of the skin should be excised, while preserving the orbicularis muscle and other connective tissue. **A.** The hollowness of eyelid is caused by a generalized inadequacy in soft tissue. **B.** The orbicularis muscle is divided 1 mm above the inferior skin incision line (gentian violet line on right eyelid). The extraneous orbicularis muscle is incorporated into the volume of the upper flap. **C.** In another case, the orbicularis muscle is divided more evenly to add bulk to both the superior and inferior flaps.

Most patients dislike pretarsal bulkiness in the upper eyelid. One exception can be made for elderly patients with thin attenuated skin and an abundance of wrinkles, in whom pretarsal fullness can appear youthful (FIGURE 2-10).

Orbital fat resection

In bulky eyelids, a small buttonhole incision is applied to the septum, through which the lateral orbital fat is partially removed. The orbital septum is a gliding membrane and is useful for preventing adhesion. Bulkiness of the medial eyelid can be addressed by excision of the medial fat. Compared to the lateral fat, the medial fat is paler, denser, and contains larger vessels, and excision of the medial fat requires more of the operator's attention for bleeding control.

Sunken eyelids with thin skin are often accompanied by bulky medial fat because the medial horn of levator aponeurosis tends to atrophy more so than the lateral horn. The medial orbital fat can be removed transconjunctivally without injuring the medial horn. Resected medial fat can be used as free graft to augment the hollow areas (FIGURE 2-11).

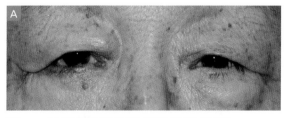
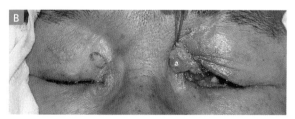
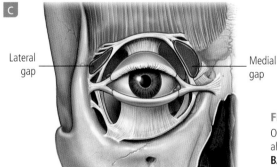

Lateral gap

Medial gap

FIGURE 2-11 • Medial bulkiness from excess fat.
Overall, the eyelid appears hollow but has a focal point of bulkiness medially. **A.** The medial horn is attenuated, resulting in bulging of the medial fat. **B.** Transconjunctival removal of the medial fat. **C.** Levator aponeurosis gap, medial and lateral gap.

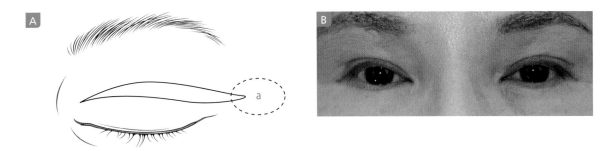

FIGURE 2-12 • **A.** Excessive removal of soft tissue towards the temporal area, 'a', can result cachectic appearance. **B.** In this patient, excessive removal of fat tissue in the the area has resulted in loss of the lateral roundness, resulting in an unnatural look.

Retro-orbicularis oculi fat (ROOF) resection

The retro-orbicularis oculi fat acts as a gliding surface between the orbicularis muscle and the orbital bone. Thus, excessive removal of ROOF over the orbital rim can result in temporary, or sometimes even permanent, adhesion and depression. This can limit free movement of levator and result in blepharoptosis. In the central or medial eyelid, resection of retro-orbicularis oculi muscle fat can cause triple fold formation. Removal of submuscular fat in the lateral eyelid is usually safe, but excessive resection can disrupt the normal convexity and should be avoided **(FIGURE 2-12)**.

Fixation

The fixation suture should be placed to the tarsal plate or the levator aponeurosis at a little higher point than upper margin of lower eyelid flap. Too high of a fixation can stretch the lower flap skin and cause deep folds and/or ectropion. At times, the lower flap can become dusky from the development of telangiectasia. In elderly patients, stretched skin appears too conspicuous and unnatural.

Elderly patients are often reluctant to have eyelid crease because of the unnatural appearance after blepharoplasty. Some operators also believe that eyelid creases cannot appear natural in elderly patients. However, a natural and aesthetically desirable eyelid creases are possible in elderly patients, provided that the low flap is not overly stretched and that the eyelid crease is without ectropion **(FIGURE 2-13)**. Beautiful eyelid creases are possible in the elderly if the operator has a competent

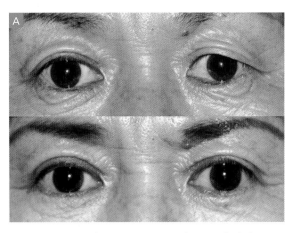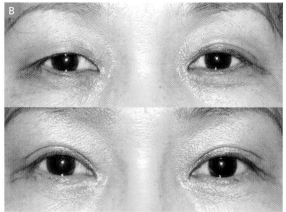

FIGURE 2-13 • Above: preoperative photographs, below: postoperative photographs.
A. Eyelid creases can appear natural even in elderly patients. **B.** The newly created eyelid crease appears just as natural as pre-existing eyelid crease.

understanding of the eyelid crease mechanism.

To prevent ectropion, depression scar and fading of the crease, the author uses the tarso-aponeurosis-orbicularis (TAO) fixation.

1. The fixation begins with the suture passing through a partial thickness of the tarsal plate at the height of the lower flap skin. The lower flap should not be outstretched.

2. The suture is then passed through the levator aponeurosis slightly above the tarsal fixation point. The distance between the tarsal fixation and the aponeurosis should be minor enough not to cause significant advancement.

3. The suture is passed through the orbicularis oculi muscle of upper border of lower flap and tied.

In elderly patients, an important consideration is whether to create the eyelid creases or simply to remove the redundant skin. A surgically created eyelid crease has the effect of making the upper eyelid skin appear less droopy and also prevents entropion. However, patients without pre-existing crease may find the eyelid crease to be highly unnatural and a significant source of self-consciousness in social settings. Also, one must consider the fact that a blepharoplasty with eyelid creases requires more recovery time than a blepharoplasty without.

In younger patients, the crease fixation is relatively deep since relapse (fading of

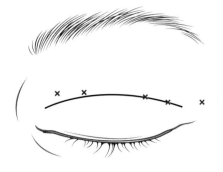

FIGURE 2-14 • Crease fixation height relative to incision line.

Relative to the incision line, the fixation should be higher in medial eyelid. This helps create a crease of uniform depth. The lateralmost fixation is made to the levator aponeurosis or the septum, since the tarsal plate does not extend to this point.

the crease) is expected to some degree. In older patients, the fixation is shallower since relapse is less common and a shallower fold is more harmonious with an elderly visage. Because the crease fixations are shallower, recovery times are less for elderly patients, compared to the recovery time required for deep folds in younger patients.

KEYPOINT 🔒

Outstretched eyelid skin in the elderly causes the following problems:

- The outstretched lower flap is associated with slight ectropion, which can be mistaken for an expression of contempt. Patients may complain about discomfort with opening the eyes.
- Because the skin is thinner, the blood vessels appear more prominent. This results in dusky texture of the skin. The pretarsal flatness can be mistaken for nervous countenance.

Location of fixation

Usually, fixations are performed at 4 to 6 locations.

- Fixations are usually placed at a lower height in elderly patients, compared to the fixation height in younger patients.
- Uniformity of crease depth can be achieved by fixing the lower flap higher medially and lower laterally, relative to the incision line (**FIGURE 2-14**).
- If the tarsal plate is large, fixation to the upper tarsal border can lead to depressed scar and ectropion.

Creating laterally extending eyelid crease

- In elderly patients, it is difficult to extend the crease beyond the lateral canthus without accurate fixation. The lateralmost fixation is made 4-6 mm beyond the lateral canthus. Since there is no tarsal plate, the suture is fixated to the levator aponeurosis or the septum. (See the section of fixation in Chapter 1.)

- The levator aponeurosis lies deeper in the lateral portion of upper eyelid **(FIGURE 2-15C)**. Fixation to the levator in the lateral eyelid may result in a crease that progressively becomes deeper until it comes to an abrupt end **(FIGURE 2-16)**. To prevent this, the lateral most fixation should be performed in a different manner. Through the lateral eyelid incision site, the oculi muscle and underlying soft tissue is opened to expose the aponeurosis. The lower margin of aponeurosis is mobilized and fixed to oculi muscle. Fixation to the lower border of aponeurosis prevents formation of deep fold. The resulting double fold is long and secure **(FIGURE 2-17A)**. The distance from the canthus to the orbital rim is longest at the raphe line. However, it becomes shorter at the upper level. The lower margin of aponeurosis is relatively mobile, and the use of this lower margin can create a long fold. As another method, the suture needle is driven 2-3 mm deep

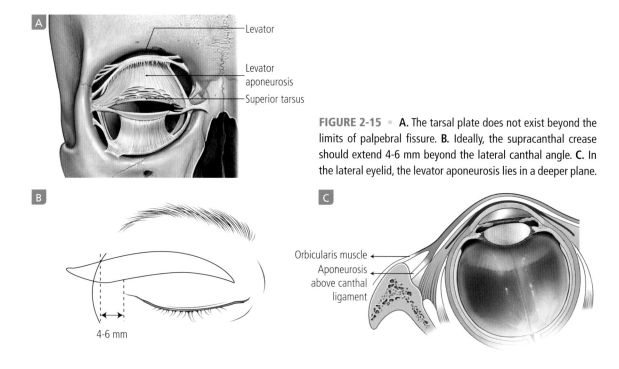

FIGURE 2-15 • **A.** The tarsal plate does not exist beyond the limits of palpebral fissure. **B.** Ideally, the supracanthal crease should extend 4-6 mm beyond the lateral canthal angle. **C.** In the lateral eyelid, the levator aponeurosis lies in a deeper plane.

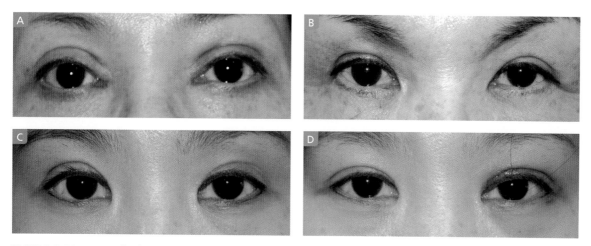

FIGURE 2-16 • Laterally, the eyelid crease can become deep and end abruptly. There is a tendency for the crease to inflect downward as well.

A. The creases end abruptly. **B.** The lateral fold heading downward. **C & D.** In the preoperative photograph, the lateral fold does not extend laterally and has an undesirable downward inflection. The creases appear more natural at postoperative day 3.

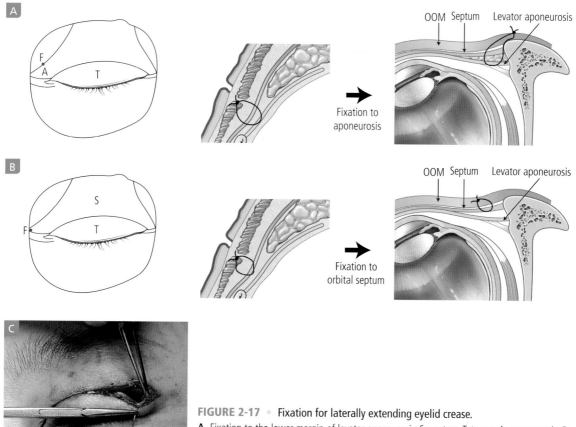

FIGURE 2-17 • Fixation for laterally extending eyelid crease.
A. Fixation to the lower margin of levator aponeurosis. S; septum, T; tarsus, A; aponeurosis, F; fixation point. **B.** Fixation to the septum nearest to the lower margin of aponeurosis. **C.** The needle is passed through the lower border of lateral aponeurosis (Method **A**). The forceps is holding onto the orbital septum, which can be used as a fixation point (Method **B**).

through the aponeurosis. Then, it is withdrawn out of the orbital rim and fixated to the orbicularis muscle. At this point, exposure of the aponeurosis or the periosteum should be avoided, as it may result in deep eyelid folds with depressed scar. Another method is fixation to the septum just near to the lower border of lateral aponeurosis **(FIGURE 2-17B)**.

 WAIT A MINUTE!

WHY DO EYELID CREASES NOT EXTEND AS EASILY IN ELDERLY PATIENTS?

In the lateral eyelid, the orbital fat descends between the septum and the aponeurosis, which worsens with aging. This descending fat interferes with the formation of crease between the levator aponeurosis and orbicularis muscle.

Direction of fixation

The lower flap should not be fixed vertically to the posterior lamella but in a radiating orientation. In the medial eyelid, the suture to the orbicularis muscle should be fixated slightly lateral to the fixation location for the tarsal plate. In the lateral eyelid, the tarsal plate should be fixed to the orbicularis muscle slightly medial **(FIGURE 2-18)**. Straight vertical fixations can result in horizontal wrinkles in the medial eyelid **(FIGURE 2-21)** and inadequate extension of the crease in the lateral eyelid.

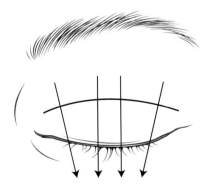

FIGURE 2-18 • Direction of fixation.
The fixation from tarsal plate to the lower flap is in a central direction.

Skin closure

Supplementary fixation suture

The permanent fixation sutures can become loose during the early recovery period due to the tension caused by edema. To minimize this risk, three or four supplementary fixation sutures can be placed to offload the tension from the permanent fixation suture. These sutures are designed to anchor the tarsal plate during skin closure. The sutures pass through skin, orbicularis muscle, tarsal plate, orbicularis muscle, and back through the skin (FIGURE 2-19). The remainder of eyelid skin is closed by a continuous suture. The skin should be everted to prevent depressed scar.

When the length is different between upper and lower incision, the temptation

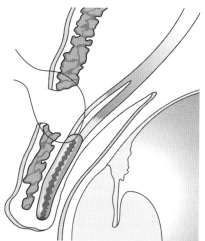

FIGURE 2-19 • Supplementary fixation suture.
At the time of skin closure, four to five sutures are placed to reduce the tension applied to the deep permanent sutures. These supplementary stitches are removed on 3rd or 4th postoperative day.

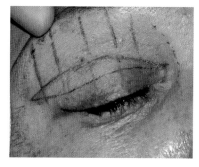 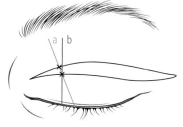 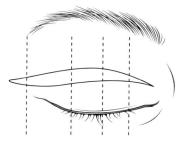

FIGURE 2-20 • Direction of skin closure.
The skin should not be closed by equal incision length (Direction 'a'). Rather, the sutures should be placed vertically (Direction 'b'). The vertical closure helps to prevent wrinkles in the medial eyelid. Thus, opening the eyelid will bring the skin of the upper and lower flap together.

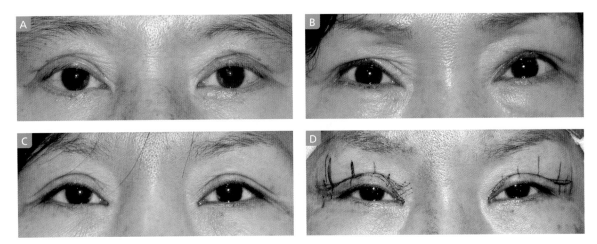

FIGURE 2-21 • Horizontal wrinkles in medial eyelid.
These horizontal wrinkles result either from absence of tarsal fixation or diagonal closure of the skin incision.

might be to close the skin by approximating points of equal length **(FIGURE 2-20A)**. However, this may lead to wrinkles in the medial eyelid **(FIGURE 2-21)**. The incisions should be closed by fixations of vertical points **(FIGURE 2-20B)**.

Usually, the eyelid skin is not undermined. However, subcutaneous dissection of the lateral eyelid can be helpful in decreasing tension and everting the skin edges.

After suture removal, skin tape is applied to the creaseless portion of the lateral eyelid for 2 weeks.

ANCILLARY PROCEDURES

Reducing recovery time

It is needless to emphasize the importance of decreasing the recovery period. To reduce the recovery time, the blepharoplasty operation should be as atraumatic as possible, as simple as possible, and the method should be one that displays little difference between immediate and final postoperative status. For example, the eyelid crease can be made with slight ectropion to account for postoperative fading of the crease. A method that creates an excessive ectropion in anticipation of significant fading of the crease tends to be associated with prolonged recovery, whereas a method that minimizes the ectropion and subsequent fading of crease will be associated with quicker recovery.

Method to reduce recovery period

The recovery time can be reduced in open blepharoplasty by minimizing trauma to the pretarsal soft tissue – a hybrid between excisional and non-incisional methods.

- First, the redundant skin is excised.
- The orbicularis muscle is resected in thick, bulky eyelids. If the eyelid is relatively hollow, the orbicularis muscle is divided and used to add volume to the upper and lower flaps.
- The pretarsal tissue should not be excised. Fullness of the pretarsal tissue is not a cause for concern. The non-incision method is used for fixation of the lower flap and the tarsal plate. Three or four stab incisions are made in the pretarsal soft tissue, which is used to introduce the tarsal fixation sutures. The lower flap should be fixated to the tarsal plate at the height that accommodates 80-90% stretch in the lower flap skin.
- The fixation should be performed between tarsal plate, aponeurosis, and orbicularis muscle (TAO fixation). The suture is driven through a partial thickness of the tarsal plate, through the aponeurosis directly superior to this point, and the orbicularis muscle anterior to the tarsal plate.

Reason behind fast recovery

- The method is atraumatic in using keyhole stab incisions for suture placement and preserves blood flow in the tissue being fixated.
- Direct fixation between the lower flap and the aponeurosis can lead to stretching of the skin, which can lead to fading of the crease and prolong recovery period. The TAO fixation incorporates both the tarsal plate and aponeurosis, which does not stretch the skin as much and requires less downtime.

Internal browpexy

Indication

Mild brow ptosis confined to the central and temporal aspect of eyebrow

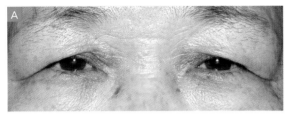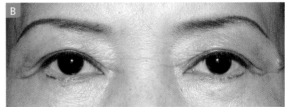

FIGURE 2-22 • **A.** Generalized hooding of the whole eyelid. **B.** The contour of the double fold is satisfactory, but the lateral portions of eyelids demonstrate noticeable skin drooping. This cannot be corrected by skin excision alone.

- Lateral brow fullness
- Unilateral brow fullness
- Prevention of brow ptosis after blepharoplasty or blepharoptosis correction

Lateral hooding can be classified into two types: generalized hooding of the whole eyelid (FIGURE 2-22A) and hooding confined to the lateral palpebral raphe (FIGURE 2-22B).

Mechanism of early lateral eyebrow ptosis

- The subbrow fat pad attachment to the periosteum is much looser in the lateral eyelid.
- The frontalis muscle lifts affects only the medial 2/3rd of the eyebrow. Lateral to the temporal crest, the lateral 1/3rd of the eyebrow is not connected to any elevating muscle (FIGURE 2-23).

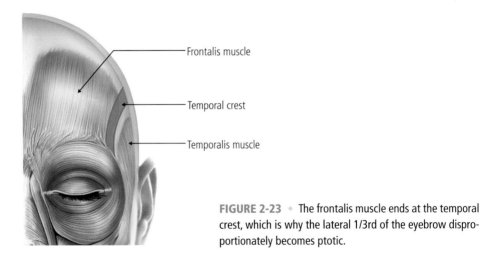

Frontalis muscle

Temporal crest

Temporalis muscle

FIGURE 2-23 • The frontalis muscle ends at the temporal crest, which is why the lateral 1/3rd of the eyebrow disproportionately becomes ptotic.

Shape of the eyebrow

In women, the eyebrows tend to have an arch shape, whereas men tend to have much flatter eyebrows. The subbrow fat pad tends to be larger in men than in women.

Postoperative brow ptosis

Brow ptosis can follow upper blepharoplasty or blepharoptosis correction because the frontalis muscle no longer needs to compensate for the levator mechanism. In such cases, excessive skin excision will only lead to more brow ptosis. The brow ptosis can lead to following problems:

- A significant excision of skin does not improve the skin redundancy.
- Crow's feet seem more accentuated in the area lateral to skin excision. This problem is not severe with sub brow blepharoplasty
- The eyelid appears more bulky. At times, the eyelid can appear even bulkier despite orbital fat resection.
- Horizontal wrinkles are formed in the medial eyelid, sometimes even across the nasal skin.

    The skin redundancy and accentuation of crow's feet can be addressed with orbicularis muscle splitting, orbicularis suspension, and internal browpexy.

Operative details for internal browpexy (FIGURE 2-24, 2-26)

1. The degree of brow ptosis is evaluated with the patient in sitting position.
2. The expected course of the supraorbital nerve is outlined.
3. The skin and orbicularis muscle are excised through a blepharoplasty incision.
4. The dissection is carried between postorbicular fascia and ROOF or between ROOF and periosteum, up 2 cm beyond the superior orbital rim.
5. Lateral brow fullness can be address by partial resection of subbrow fat.
6. The subbrow orbicularis muscle and the ROOF are anchored to the periosteum about 1-1.5 cm above the orbital rim. The lateral third of the eyebrow is the highest point of the arch, which usually corresponds with the location of lateral limbus.

During the dissection of preperiosteal space, care must be taken not to injure the deep branch of the supraorbital nerve, which comes out of the supraorbital foramen

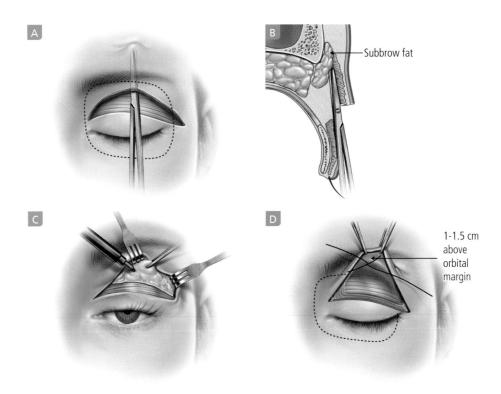

FIGURE 2-24 • Internal browpexy.
A & B. The supraperiosteal space is dissected. **C.** If necessary, the subbrow fat (ROOF) is removed. **D.** The orbicularis oculi muscle is anchored to the periosteum.

and runs superolaterally until it meets and runs 5-10 mm inside along the temporal crest. At the orbital rim, it runs in the supraperiosteal space and perforates through the deep galea about 3 cm above the orbital rim **(FIGURE 2-25)**. Because of this anatomy, the safe plane of dissection is between the orbicularis fascia and the subbrow fat. Also, one must avoid dissecting too deeply beneath the subbrow fat.

Orbicularis muscle splitting

Efficacy

1. Prevention of brow ptosis – The orbicularis muscle depresses the eyebrow and disrupting this muscle has the effect of decreasing the depressing force.
2. Improvement to crow's feet.
3. Insertion of fat tissue prevents re-adhesion between divided ends of the

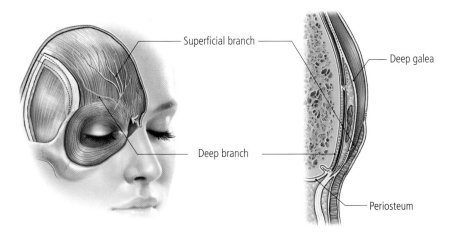

FIGURE 2-25 • The deep branch of supraorbital nerve.
The branch runs superolaterally until it meets and runs 5-10 mm inside along the temporal crest. At the orbital rim, it runs in the supraperiosteal space and perforates through the deep galea about 3 cm above the orbital rim.

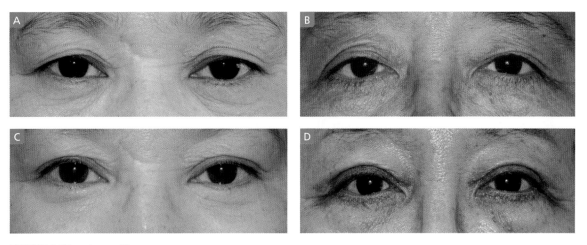

FIGURE 2-26 • Internal browpexy cases.
Internal browpexy was performed in anticipation of the brow ptosis following senile blepharoplasty.

orbicularis muscle. This prevents depression in the contour from the muscle division.

4. The lateral orbital fat often interferes with crease formation. Mobilization of this fat promotes crease formation in the lateral eyelid.

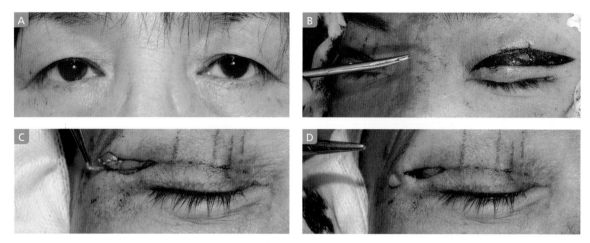

FIGURE 2-27 • Orbicularis muscle splitting.
A. Preoperative photo of a patient with lateral hooding and prominent crow's feet. **B.** After skin excision, a strip of orbicularis oculi muscle is resected along the length of the desired crease (4-6 mm beyond the lateral raphe). Lateral to the end of resection, the orbicularis muscle is further divided using electrocautery without any removal of muscle mass. **C.** The lateral fat is mobilized prior to being inserted between the divided edges of the muscle. **D.** A pull-out suture is used to secure the orbital fat in its new location.

Operative detail

- Open blepharoplasty: The skin and orbicularis muscle are excised.
- The orbicularis muscle is further divided in the lateral direction beyond the existing skin incision. This can be achieved by undermining the skin then using the electrocautery to divide the orbicularis muscle. During this step, care must be taken not to injure the frontal branch of the facial nerve.

The lateral orbital fat is mobilized and inserted into the space between the divided orbicularis muscles. The amount of inserted fat should be appropriate for the space, and surplus fat is excised. The mobilized fat is fixated in the space using a pullout fixation suture (FIGURE 2-27).

The division of orbicularis muscle can lead to either depression of the contour or re-adhesion of the divided orbicularis muscle. The insertion of the lateral fat into the divided space prevents both of these potential problems. The orbicularis suspension can augment this method.

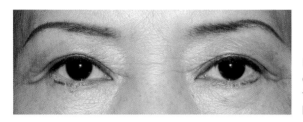

FIGURE 2-28 • In this patient, the eyelid creases appear natural except for the lateral hooding, which cannot be addressed by skin excision alone.

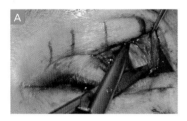 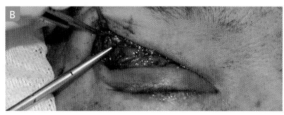

FIGURE 2-29 • **A.** The dissection is carried superiorly in the plane below the ROOF. **B.** The orbicularis muscle is fixated to the periosteum.

Orbicularis suspension

Orbicularis suspension is a method that counteracts postoperative brow ptosis while still addressing lateral hooding. The method is similar to internal browpexy, but the anchoring point is lower. Hooding over lateral palpebral raphe represents disproportionate drooping of the redundant skin. Large excision of the skin over the raphe area does not solve the problem and promote postoperative brow ptosis **(FIGURE 2-28, 2-34)**.

Operative detail (FIGURE 2-29)

- Orbicularis oculi muscle is divided.
- The dissection is carried superiorly in the retro-orbital space. The dissection can extended further superiorly to accommodate for internal browpexy, if needed.
- The orbicularis muscle, along with posterior fascia and ROOF, are lifted and fixated to the periosteum.

During the suspension of orbicularis muscle to the periosteum, adjusting the tension of fixation to a proper degree is important above all else. The orbicularis muscle should be fixated to the periosteum at the height of the eyebrow in the supine position **(FIGURE 2-30, 2-31)**. Excessive elevation can lead to dimpling and/or

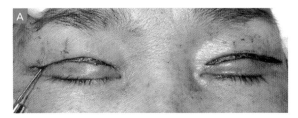 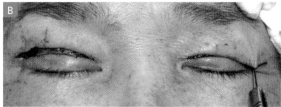

FIGURE 2-30 • **A.** Orbicularis suspension had been performed for the right side in this photograph. With the patient in supine position, the orbicularis oculi muscle and the periosteum were fixated at the same height. The upper flap does not easily descend when pulled downward. **B.** Prior to orbicularis suspension, the left side can easily be pulled downward.

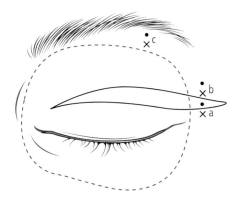

FIGURE 2-31 • Various anchor points for orbicularis suspension.
Orbicularis, postorbicularis fascia, and ROOF are anchored to the periosteum. At each location, the orbicularis oculi muscle (marked with 'x') is fixated to the point above (marked by '•').
(a) Orbicularis oculi of the lower flap.
(b) Orbicularis oculi of the upper flap.
(c) Subbrow orbicularis oculi muscle (internal browpexy).

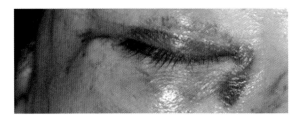

FIGURE 2-32 • An example of dimpling after orbicularis oculi suspension.

buckling of the skin **(FIGURE 2-32)**. These problems are not apparent in the supine position, and intraoperative examination should be performed in the sitting position for this reason. Wrinkling over the lateral raphe can also be evaluated by gently pulling down on the eyebrow **(FIGURE 2-33)**.

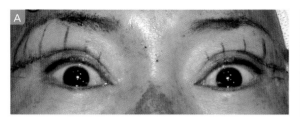
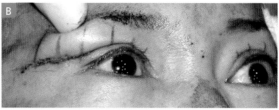

FIGURE 2-33 • Immediate postoperative photograph after orbicularis muscle suspension. No wrinkles can be observed over the lateral raphe despite depression of the eyebrow.

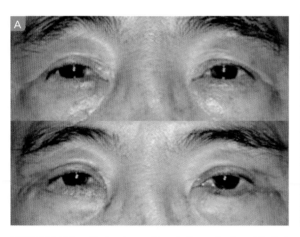
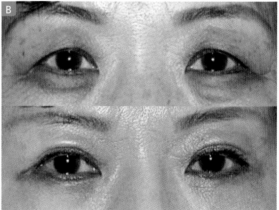

FIGURE 2-34 • Pre/postoperative photographs for orbicularis oculi suspension.
Above: The drooping of eyelid over the lateral raphe is distinct. Below: The operation has corrected the lateral drooping in both patients.

Complications of

- Edema: The wide dissection can cause severe edema.
- Temporary hypoesthesia: This can be cause by manipulation or injury to the deep branch of supraorbital nerve.
- Dimpling: The level of elevation must be adequate to avoid dimpling.
- High crease
- Limitation of eyebrow motility: This can occur from the anchoring being too tight.

MISCELLANEOUS ISSUES

Senile blepharoptosis

Blepharoptosis can be caused by aging, previous blepharoplasty, and thyroid diseases. Contact lens use has become a frequent cause in the past two decades.

Blepharoptosis is caused by dehiscence or disinsertion of the levator aponeurosis. The problem can be addressed by advancement of the aponeurosis alone or of aponeurosis and Muller's muscle together. This topic will be further discussed in the section on blepharoptosis.

Pre-existing eyelid crease is satisfactory, but the eyelid has lateral hooding

If the existing crease is desirable, subbrow lifting alone may be an appropriate solution or it can be performed in conjunction with blepharoplasty. The need for crease fixation is questionable in the presence of pre-existing crease. The blepharoplasty incision can disrupt the innate eyelid creases. If the crease becomes faint or disappears after the incision, then crease fixation is a necessary. If the incision has disconnected the lower flap, then buried fixation sutures are necessary. Usually, this is not the case, and some adhesion remains to the lower flap. As such, four supplementary fixation sutures are sufficient in allowing the lower flap to re-adhere during the recovery period (FIGURE 2-35A). These sutures are used for the following reasons:

- The adhesion tissue may have been removed with excision of the scar.
- It is possible for an extra crease to develop in the upper flap (triple fold). To reduce the risk of this happening, the supplementary sutures can be used to remove the degree of freedom in the upper flap (FIGURE 2-35A).

The supplementary suture should incorporate the orbicularis muscle and tarsal plate into the skin closure for prevention of depressed scar.

If the height of crease is desirable, the fixation should follow the original crease line. However, this represents an opportunity to change the shape and height of the crease if the patient wishes to do so.

Skin laxity of the lower flap can be addressed during the operation as well. The incision is made below the pre-existing crease with a strip excision of the skin. The

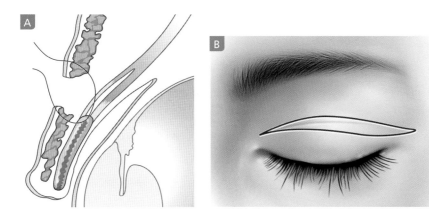

FIGURE 2-35 •

Supplementary fixation suture.
A. With a pre-existing crease, this temporary fixation of skin, orbicularis muscle, and tarsal plate is sufficient in maintaining the crease. Lack of any such fixation may lead to extraneous creases (triple fold). **B.** Skin laxity of the lower flap can be addressed by skin excision and resetting the crease line at a lower height.

lower flap skin is stretched about 80% of the full length, while the crease remains in its prior height **(FIGURE 2-35B)**.

Senile blepharoplasty without an eyelid crease

At times, a patient may present with severe redundancy of the eyelid skin but wishes not to have an eyelid crease after the operation. This is especially common for male patients without pre-existing eyelid crease. The following strategies can decrease the risk of crease formation.

- The inferior incision line is placed low, at 3-5 mm above the ciliary margin. The eyelid creases do not easily form so close to the eyelid margin, or if they form, are usually temporary. If the incision is too low, however, the risk of scar formation is high from discrepancies in skin thickness of the upper and lower flap.
- Soft tissue removal should be minimize to prevent unwanted crease formation.
- The gap should be minimized between the divided edges of the orbicularis muscle. The skin should be closed with adequate eversion, using vertical mattress.
- Skin bandage should be used over the incision line after suture removal.

The problem with skin excision is that the upper eyelid becomes bulky due to the descent of eyebrow. This is especially the case in men with thicker eyelid skin. In senile blepharoplasty, the eyelid can appear to be even bulkier than prior to operation, despite a significant excision of soft tissue. Because of this, even more soft tissue may need to be removed, which can promote the formation of unwanted

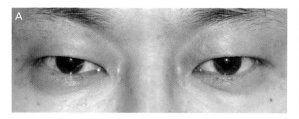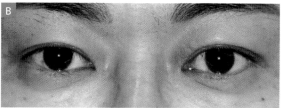

FIGURE 2-36 • This male patient wished for a relatively discrete eyelid rejuvenation. The resulting low crease (inside fold) was an acceptable solution for the patient.

creases. To avoid this crease formation, the author usually recommends a low eyelid crease (AKA inside fold). Inner folds are often acceptable to patients who do not wish for eyelid creases. Compared to eyelids without crease, this approach decreases the recurrence of skin hooding **(FIGURE 2-36)**.

Senile ectropion in upper lid

Senile ectropion is due to atrophy of soft tissue and often accompanies blepharoptosis. Correction of blepharoptosis is often followed by dry eye syndrome, which can be explained by two mechanisms. The first mechanism is the discomfort caused by direct drying of the grey line by ectropion. This can be demonstrated by causing temporary ectropion with an eyelid stylus. Second, the keratinization of the grey line leads to closure of the orifice of meibomian gland. This subsequently leads to thinning of the lipid layer, without which the aqueous and mucinous layer of the tear film quickly evaporates. Fortunately, the orifice closure from keratinization is a reversible change and can be resolved with correction of ectropion. This issue is extensively discussed in Chapter 3.

INFRABROW BLEPHAROPLASTY

Infrabrow blepharoplasty remedies many of the disadvantages of conventional blepharoplasty.

Differences between infrabrow and conventional blepharoplasty

Because of the incision over the crease line, conventional blepharoplasty can easily change the shape of the crease line, which is sometimes undesirable to many patients. In contrast, infrabrow blepharoplasty only removes the redundant skin without involving the crease line, and the eyelid crease is restored to original shape. The operation also requires less recovery time.

The disadvantages of infrabrow blepharoplasty are that it cannot control the eyelid crease and that fat removal is not an option for bulky eyes. To address the former problem, the eyelid crease can be created or manipulated by an additional operation. This double-prong approach to blepharoplasty allows partial resections of the excessive skin through two separate incisions, which lowers the risk of complications that can arise for larger excisions in a single operative site (e.g. elongation of scar, lateral hooding, and accentuation of crow's feet). Another disadvantage of this operation is eyebrow ptosis and flatness. To prevent brow ptosis, the edge of orbicularis muscle is fixed to the frontalis muscle or the periosteum of frontalis bone. Also, this is contraindicated if the eyebrow is lower than the orbital rim itself or if the risk of postoperative brow ptosis is high.

Conventional blepharoplasty can suffer from a discrepancy in skin thickness between upper and lower flaps. This discrepancy is much less with infrabrow blepharoplasty because the skin excision do not cross the unit boundary of upper eyelid skin.

Also, the conventional blepharoplasty incision can lead to aggravation of crow's feet over the lateral orbital rim. With infrabrow blepharoplasty, the incision is father away from this area and does not contribute to formation of crow's feet.

Indications

- Dermatochalasis in patients who do not want eyelid creases or do not want changes to pre-existing creases
- Thick eyebrows – the partial excision of lower brow can be incorporated.
- Excision of scar from previous infrabrow blepharoplasty
- High eyebrows
- Tattooed eyebrows
- Patients who require the quickest recovery period possible

Operative detail

- Design and skin excision
- Orbicularis muscle excision
- Orbicularis muscle suspension.
- Closure

Design and skin excision

- The skin excision is designed below the eyebrow. The locations are marked for supraorbital nerve and the supratrochlear nerve located 1 cm medially from the supraorbital nerve.
- If the eyebrows have tattoo, the excision design should be performed according to the shape of the tattoo. If the eyebrow or the tattoo is too thick, the design can incorporate either the brow or the tattooed skin for a brow-lifting effect. This can also help to hide the incision scar into the border of tattoo or eyebrow. It is important not to injure the follicular bed.
- The amount of skin excision should be determined by the method described earlier for upper blepharoplasty.
- Usually, dermatochalasis is more noticeable in the lateral eyelid, and as such, incisions frequently begin at the supraorbital nerve. If the skin drooping is significant toward the medial eyelid, the incision can be extended medially. However, the incision should be limited to the skin and the muscle left intact, to avoid injuring the nerve.
- Laterally, the excision is extended all the way to the end of either the eyebrow or the tattooed skin.
- The skin is excised according to the design.

Dissection and excision of orbicularis oculi muscle

- A strip of orbicularis oculi muscle is excised following skin removal. The muscle, however, should not be excised near the supra-orbital nerve and the supra-trochlear nerve. Additionally, the orbicularis muscle is not excised in the sunken eyelid. Rather, it should be turned over to add bulkiness to the eyelid.

- The dissection is carried superiorly subgaleal layer below to exposure the perios-teum and confirm the deep branch of supraorbital nerve. This dissection plane helps to promote adhesion and is more secure than the plane beneath the sub-brow fat. Some argue that sub-muscular dissection leads to immobilization of the eyebrow and that subbrow fat yields a more natural eyebrow. With the latter, the adhesions are not secure.

- In the inferior flap, the dissection is performed superficially and deep to the orbicularis oculi muscle. The mobilized muscle flap is anchored to the perios-teum or frontalis muscle 2 to 3 mm above the superior flap margin. This step is optional, however.

- The subcutaneous layer is closed. When closing the skin, it is better to start the sutures in both ends to minimize the risk of dog ear formation **(FIGURE 2-37, 2-38)**.

Complications

- Dysesthesia
- Scar
- Loss of eyebrow arch

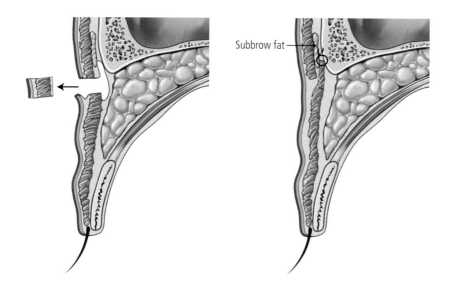

Subbrow fat

FIGURE 2-37 •

Subbrow lifting.
The lower flap is secured to the periosteum or the frontalis muscle.

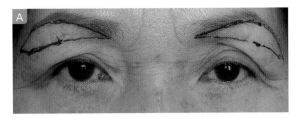
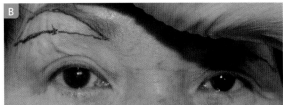
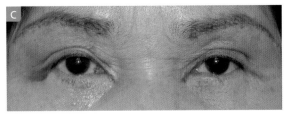

FIGURE 2-38 • Subbrow lifting.
A. Incision design. **B.** The skin excision is designed while simulating the appearance of the postoperative eyelid by elevating the eyebrow manually. **C.** Postoperative outcome.

KEYPOINT

In aging blepharoplasty

1. The eyelid incision should be designed while partially stretching the eyelid skin. In the same manner, the lower flap should be fixated to the tarsal plate in a partially stretched state, as to allow some wrinkling in the lower flap skin. In other words, the lower flap should not be fixated too high on the tarsal plate.
2. The lower flap should neither be undermined nor its muscle resected.
3. The pretarsal soft tissue should not be removed. The fixation sutures can be introduced via stab incisions made in the pretarsal tissue.
4. To avoid the disadvantages of low fixations on the tarsal plate, the fixation can incorporate levator aponeurosis above the tarsal plate. (Tarsus-aponeurosis-orbicularis fixation)
5. Excessive skin resections are to be avoided. In patients with severe chalasis, the orbicularis oculi muscle can be excised to help reduce the bulk of the upper flap.

The information in the following section is shared with the patient after an operation:

THINGS TO KEEP IN MIND AFTER UPPER EYELID SURGERY

Postoperative changes

The following can be worrisome in the postoperative period: swelling, bruise, height and depth of crease, and the appearance of scars. Bruises will usually disappear within two weeks of surgery, but the remaining items will take 3 to 6 months to improve. At times, some of these problems may last for up to a year, depending on individual factors.

Edema

As edema subsides, the bulkiness in pretarsal area will improve. The time required for resolution of edema varies depending on the operation and individual factors. Usually, the edema resolves faster for lower creases.

Depth

Initially, the crease may appear too conspicuous and deeply folded, with everted eyelashes. However, the crease will become more faint with time, and the ectropion will become more neutral (3-6 months).

Scar

In the first month, the scar can appear erythematous and feel indurated. The erythema and induration will decrease over a 3 to 6 month period but can last longer in some individuals.

Postoperative instructions

1. The suture is usually removed on the 3rd postoperative day, or half of the sutures can be removed on 2nd day with the remaining sutures removed on the 4th day.
2. The face can be washed using soap the day after suture removal. Lathering of the eyelids should be gentle.
3. Cool compress is applied for the first two days after the operation, which reduces edema and bruising. The compress is not helpful after suture removal. If the risk of triple fold formation is high, cool compress should not applied on the first

day to allow the eyelids to be open as much as possible.

4. Cosmetic products may be applied 1 week after surgery. Warm compress can be applied after the first 2 weeks. The usual cool compress can be used as warm compress by submerging it in hot water prior to application. Warm compress helps to resolve edema and bruises by increasing circulation, but this is not essential.

5. The following should be avoided for the first month: alcohol, tobacco, vigorous exercise, sauna.

6. Medications may be prescribed for patients with history of hypertrophic scars or for secondary operations.

7. Rubbing or frequent palpation of the eyelid should be avoided in the first 2-3 weeks can lead to dehiscence or widening of the scar.

📑 REFERENCES

1. Flowers RS : Blepharoplasty and periorbital aesthetic surgery. Clin Plast Surg 20;193-207, 1993.
2. Baek BS, Park DH : Cosmetic and reconstructive oculoplastic surgery. 3rd Edition, Seoul Koonja Publishung Company, 2009.

SECONDARY UPPER BLEPHAROPLASTY

- Scars
- Depth problems including loss of fold
- Height problems
- Pretarsal fullness
- Asymmetry
- Multiple creases (triple folds)
- Sunken eyelid/primary triple fold
- Blepharoptosis
- Removal of the eyelid fold
- Conclusion

Aesthetic standards for eyelids vary across ethnic groups and cultures. While a certain contemporary aesthetic standard may be satisfactory to large numbers of patients, complications after double eyelid operations are specific to each individual patient. As such, the only approach that is universal in the management of double eyelid complications is this: only with proper recognition of the underlying etiology can a surgeon offer and execute the solution to the complaint each patient brings.

In this chapter, we discuss a list of the most complaints after a double eyelid operation. For each complication, we identify the underlying problem of the index operation and present the solution developed over the course of the senior author's career as an oculoplastic surgeon.

SCARS

Eyelid skin does not develop hypertrophic response in most cases. When hypertrophic response is observed after an eyelid operation, the fundamental problem could be that the patient just has a tendency to scar. In many instances, however, the problem is not with the patient but with the surgeon who has performed the index operation.

The most common technical mistake is the lack of understanding behind the distribution of superior-posterior force vector of levator muscle unequally distributed between the inferior and superior skin flaps (FIGURE 3-1). A less forgivable mistake is to leave sutures out for more than 5 days; epithelial tunnels form around sutures only 7 days after operation. Delayed removal of sutures should never be a cause for hypertrophic scars after double eyelid operation.

In younger patients with robust eyelid mechanisms, the incisions do not have to be extended along the full length of eyelid to create a fold of desired length. A shorter incision is usually sufficient to create the wanted fold.

A clear distinction must be made between a wide scar and a depressed scar. A wide scar is a problem of the skin itself, whereas depressed scars result from changes in the underlying connective tissue such as excessive removal of the orbicularis muscle (FIGURE 3-2) and deep crease (FIGURE 3-3).

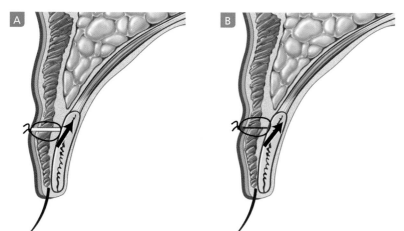

FIGURE 3-1 •

A. Immediately after fixation. **B.** A few days after operation. Repeated opening of the eyelid results in dislocation of the lower flap.

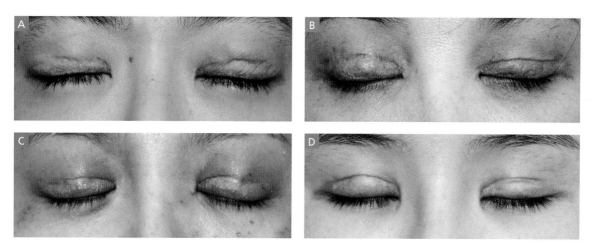

FIGURE 3-2 • Depressed scar results from excision of pretarsal oculi muscle.

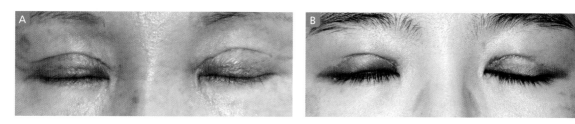

FIGURE 3-3 • Depressed scar in the ectropion.

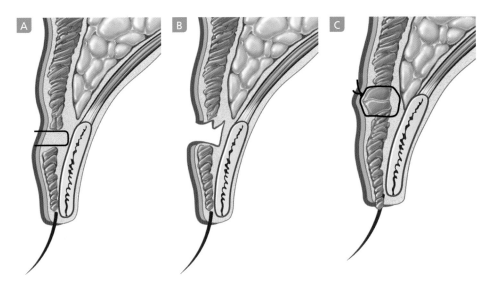

FIGURE 3-4 • Correction of depressed scar.
A. Excision of the skin containing the scar tissue. **B.** After excision of scar tissue. **C.** The skin and oculi muscle are approximated.

Scar revision

An eyelid scar revision must obey wound healing principles that govern all aspects of surgical incision management. The operation must remain as aseptically possible. The surgeon and instrument, both, must be atraumatic with the eyelid tissue. All layers – not just skin - should be approximated with as little tension as possible.

Scar excision and re-approximation of the skin does nothing to address problems of depressed scar. The missing strip of orbicularis oculi must be reconstructed by undermining and advancing the remaining muscle edge from the upper flap (FIGURE 3-4). Such undermining is also beneficial if the normal skin is inverted next to the scar. For skin suture, interrupted suture can place perpendicular tension, leaves better scar, but takes additional time. Simple continuous suture can place diagonal tension. The author prefers interlocking continuous suture as it applies the same amount of tension as interrupted sutures while saving valuable operative time.

DEPTH PROBLEMS INCLUDING LOSS OF FOLD

All surgically created eyelid folds soften during the first few months following operation. The crease may eventually be too deep, too shallow, or disappear altogether. The degree to which these changes occur is determined by patient characteristics and surgical technique.

Patient factors associated with postoperative changes to eyelid crease are 1) thick skin and abundant soft tissue, 2) blepharoptosis, 3) sunken eyelid, 4) enopthalmos, 5) previous history of failed double eyelid operation, 6) younger age, 7) low-lying preoperative crease, 8) presence of epicanthal fold, and 9) extreme weight gain.

Technical factors which increase the chance of relapse/fixation failure are 1) inaccurate approximation of connective tissue, 2) insufficient preparation of the tarsal plate fixation point, 3) low fixation, and 4) loosening of the fixation due to hematoma or edema. Low fixation points may create supratarsal folds which are too low. Inadequate soft tissue removal above the tarsal plate can prevent close approximation of the connective tissue as well as bunching of fat tissue into the loop of suture holding the muscle to the tarsal plate. The presence of fat tissue within the suture loop can introduce mechanical redundancy with expansion from edema and/or hematoma and subsequent disappearance of the surgically created crease.

Fold-resistant eyelid

The resistance of an eyelid against the maintenance of skin crease is estimated at the preoperative consultation. Fold-resistant eyelids tend to require significantly more force when using the eyelid stylus and the created fold disappears rather quickly when compared to eyelids which maintain postoperative creases without significant changes.

Patient factors which predict high resistance to fold formation include thick skin, abundant soft tissue, blepharoptosis, highly elastic skin in younger patients, sunken eyelids, enophthalmos, history of failed double eyelid operation, and adhered lower flap. Eyelids with epicanthal folds show high resistance along the medial side. Though this is not a preoperative patient factor, weight gain in the intermediate postoperative period can precipitate loss of surgically created fold.

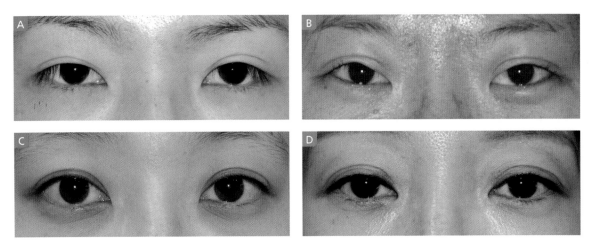

FIGURE 3-5 • Two types of shallow folds.
A & B. Drooping of lower skin flap. **C & D.** Wrinkles in the lower flap.

Preventing loss of surgically created fold

To prevent relapse, avoid intrusion of soft tissue between the levator aponeurosis and dermis or the orbicularis muscle while tying the suture. If a patient has fold-resistant eyelids, it is important to create a fold that is deep enough to result in a slight ectropion with the expectation that it will subside. At this juncture, controlling the depth of the fold is of utmost importance. If the created fold is too deep, this slight ectropion may remain even if the fold becomes shallower over time.

Correction of shallow crease

At times, there is fat or connective tissue between the skin and levator aponeurosis or between either of those and the tarsal plate. This is especially the case for the medial side of upper eyelid, where the pretarsal fat is abundant. Inadequate clearance between these points can easily lead to fixation failure. If blepharoptosis or epicanthal fold is recognized, it must be dealt with first to reduce resistance. In case of a relapsed eyelid, the adhesion beneath the crease must be released because the adhesion from the lower flap will interfere with the newly created fold. In patients whose eyelid skin lacks the elasticity after the previous operation, the newly created fold should be deeper than usual to prevent another relapse **(FIGURE 3-6)**.

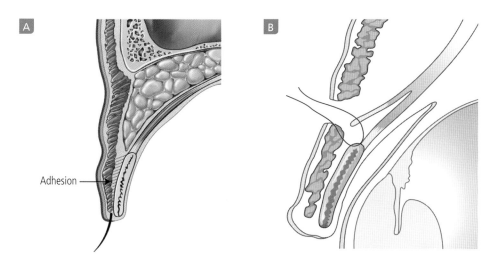

FIGURE 3-6 • Correction of shallow fold.
A. If present, adhesion of lower flap requires dissection. **B.** The oculi muscle of lower flap is fixated at a high point on the aponeurosis.

Deep crease or ectropion

High fixations may result in deep folds and ectropion. The everted eyelids imbue the rest of face with an aggressive appearance, and a depressed scar is visible when the eyes are closed. Patient may complain of a tugging sensation in the eyelids. The palpebral fissure may become larger or may become paradoxically smaller if the folds are extremely deep. The skin just above the fold tends to bulge.

High fixations inadvertently increase the palpebral fissure because the levator aponeurosis is plicated when the lower flap is fixed at a high point on levator aponeurosis. In case of severe ectropion, the mucous membrane is exposed. The mucocutaneous junction becomes keratinized - leading to dry eye syndrome.

Correction

The first step in correcting the fold depth is to release the adhesions amongst orbicularis oculi muscle, levator aponeurosis, tarsal plate, and/or the dermis. If this first manipulation resolves ectropion, fixating the lower flap to a more inferior location is sufficient. If not, the lower flap must be undermined and secured onto the lower tarsus (redraping procedure).

The second step is to taken to prevent another complication of secondary eyelid operations – the formation of triple folds. The surgeon must take care not to allow a

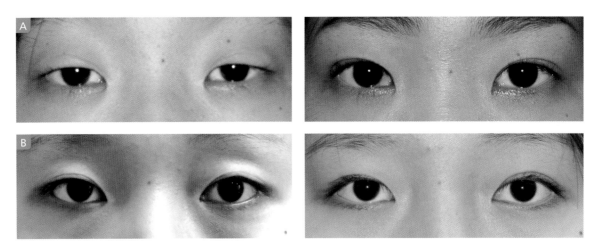

FIGURE 3-7 • Before and after shallow fold correction.
A. Complete loss of fold. **B.** Shallow fold.

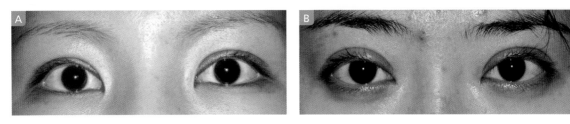

FIGURE 3-8 • **A.** Low and deep fold. **B.** High and deep fold.

new adhesion from forming in the previous fold location by introducing the orbital fat and septum into the space between the aponeurosis and the orbicularis muscle.

Deep crease is often accompanied by high fold, and the operations to correct these two features are very similar. The only significant difference between the two correction methods is that the location of the previous crease is maintained in cases of deep crease without high fold and that the new crease is designed lower than that of the previous crease and the skin in between is excised in cases of high fold alone. Correction of deep crease will be described again along with correction of high fold in the following section.

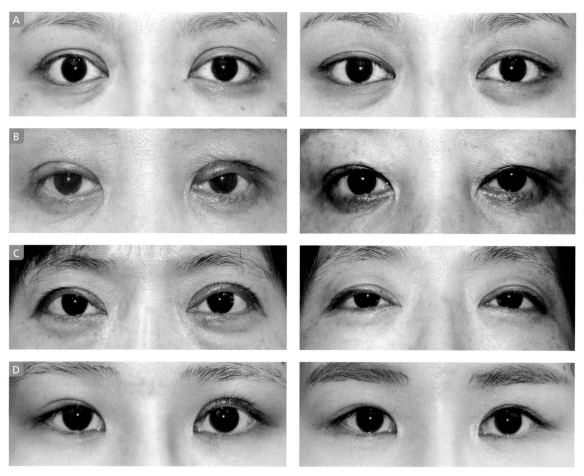

FIGURE 3-9 • Before and after correction of ectropion.

HEIGHT PROBLEMS

Low fold

Low fold refers to eyelids displaying dissatisfactory small width below the crease. Usually this is because of a low design, but at times a low fold may be formed from a shallow fold, making the fold seem lower than expected **(FIGURE 3-10)**. Aside from that, it may appear in an eyelid with redundant skin, when not excised sufficiently.

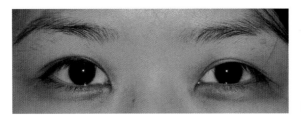

FIGURE 3-10 • Low fold.

Correcting a low fold

There are three approaches to correcting a low fold. The first is an open blepharoplasty by which the skin and orbicularis muscle is excised above the previous crease. The second is a closed double eyelid operation (sutureless or minimal incision) that creates a mechanically overriding crease above the previous crease. The third is a combination of the soft-tissue excision and mechanical fixation (FIGURE 3-11).

The first approach (open blepharoplasty) can incorporate scar revision and allows for excision of redundant skin in older patients. However, the surgeon must be cautious to leave enough eyelid skin as to minimize the risk of post blepharoplasty brow ptosis. In patients without significant redundancy of eyelid skin, excision of orbicularis muscle above the old crease is more important than excision of the skin. Maximal elevation of eyebrows should result in 80-90% elevation of upper eyelid margin in patients with appropriate skin excision. This can be used as a preoperative demonstration to the patient (FIGURE 3-11A). This method allows for increasing the crease height for redundant eyelid skin but is limited in those eyelids without skin redundancy.

The second approach (tarsal fixation) allows considerable elevation of the fold crease but will create for an additional scar, if secondary incisions were necessary. This approach is more appropriate for patients who have inconspicuous scars from the first operation and wish for the eyelid fold to be higher. If the previous fold is strongly defined (i.e. too deep), a simple mechanical fixation may result in multiple eyelid folds. To minimize such risk, the lower flap can be undermined through a small incision window. This can significantly attenuate the primary fold to a faint appearance. Patients should be warned of the potential for pretarsal fullness from the scar tissue after the initial operation (FIGURE 3-11B).

The combined approach of open blepharoplasty and mechanical fixation is

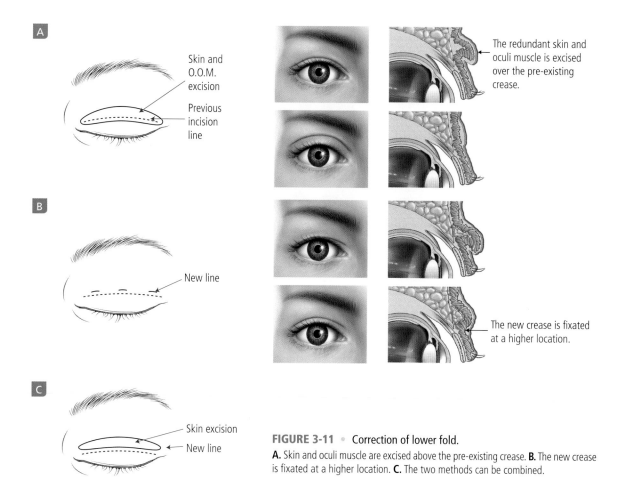

FIGURE 3-11 • Correction of lower fold.
A. Skin and oculi muscle are excised above the pre-existing crease. **B.** The new crease is fixated at a higher location. **C.** The two methods can be combined.

reserved for patients with very low folds and great redundancy in eyelid skin (**FIGURE 3-11C**).

High creases

In many East Asian cultures, high eyelid fold is a facial feature associated with aggressiveness and antagonistic personal attitude. Clinically, patients complain of unnatural appearance, depressed scar, and excessive eversion of eyelashes. It is almost always accompanied by a pretarsal fullness that does not improve with time and also is often associated with minimal blepharoptosis. In the latter case, the skin adhered to the levator aponeurosis and prevents recursion of the muscle.

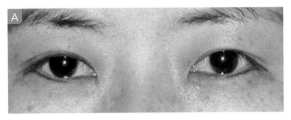
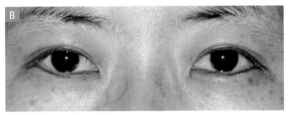

FIGURE 3-12 • The soft tissue excision method **(FIGURE 3-11A)** was used to correct the low folds in this patient.

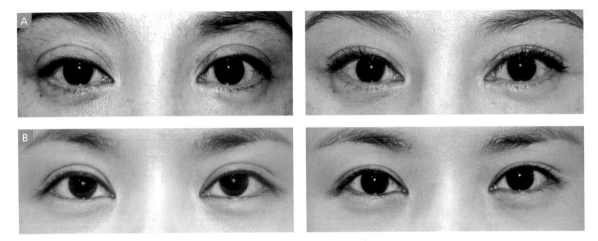

FIGURE 3-13 • Correction of high fold. Before and after surgery.

Causes

High creases can be caused by high incision lines, high fixation, excessive skin excision, unintended adhesion, blepharoptosis, or sunken eyelid **(FIGURE 3-14)**. Among these factors, the most common cause is too high of an incision line during the initial operation **(FIGURE 3-13A)**. Fixation of the lower flap to a high point can result in high folds with eversion of eyelashes **(FIGURE 3-13B)**. The problem can also result from excessive skin resection, which leaves insufficient skin to cover the crease. Patients with blepharoptosis tend to develop high folds after eyelid fold operations which does not address the mechanical etiology behind the ptosis.

High creases can be observed with deep, normal, or shallow fold depths. The most common form type is a fold that is both high and deep, which is often accompanied by ectropion. At times, patients might have folds of varying depth. (i.e. a fold that is shallow in the medial side but deep over the pupils.)

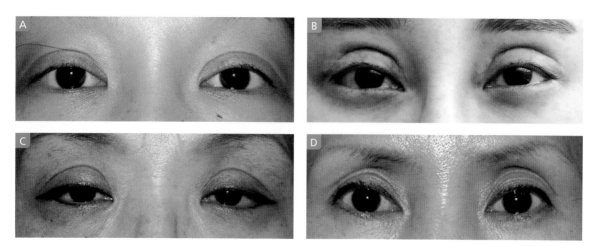

FIGURE 3-14 • High folds with varying etiology.
A. High incision from prior operation. **B.** High fixation. **C.** Ptosis. **D.** Sunken eyelid.

Correction of high creases

As with all things, high creases should be corrected according to the cause (FIGURE 3-15). Generally, the secondary operation incorporates an open blepharoplasty with skin excision. The upper margin of this excision is along the fold that is to be revised, and the lower margin marks the new fold height. If the skin lacks redundancy and lagopthalmos is expected, skin is not resected. Rather, a lower incision can be used to undermine the upper flap and release the high fold (FIGURE 3-17).

Releasing the fold through the preaponeurotic layer minimizes the risk of re-adhesion because it is the deeper layer. In patients with blepharoptosis, this deeper dissection plane is a natural choice, as this is the plane of dissection needed to address the levator mechanism. For the same reason, however, this plane of dissection can injure the levator aponeurosis and result in postoperative blepharoptosis. In contrast, releasing through the preseptal layer minimizes this risk, but is associated with increased risk for triple fold formation.

High crease with ectropion of upper eyelid

High fixations may result in deep folds and ectropion. The everted eyelids imbue the rest of face with an aggressive appearance, and a depressed scar is visible when the eyes are closed. Patient may complain of a tugging sensation in the eyelids. The skin just above the fold tends to bulge.

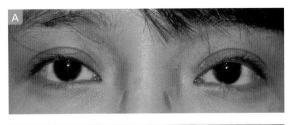
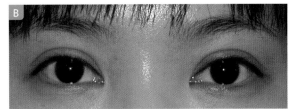
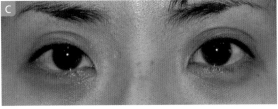

FIGURE 3-15 • Various manifestations of high fold.
A. High fold with ectropion. **B.** High fold with normal depth. **C.** High and shallow fold.

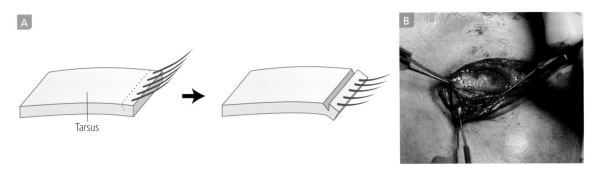

Tarsus

FIGURE 3-16 • Scoring incision of tarsus.
A. The tarsal plate is scored to correct ectropion. **B.** Intraoperative view of the scored tarsal plate.

In case of severe ectropion, the mucous membrane is exposed. The mucocutaneous junction becomes keratinized - leading to dry eye syndrome.

Ectropion can be addressed by the following 3 steps

The second step should be taken into consideration to prevent another complication of secondary eyelid operations – the formation of triple folds and recurrence of ectropion. The surgeon must take care not to allow a new adhesion from forming in the previous fold location by introducing the orbital fat and septum into the space between the aponeurosis and the orbicularis muscle and orbicularis muscle enforcement

- Step 1 (Adhesiolyis): Adhesion is released in the pre-aponeurotic plane. If this first manipulation resolves ectropion, fixating the lower flap to a more inferior location is sufficient. However, the fold may become deeper despite adequate release in the upper flap. In such case, the lower flap is also contributing to the fold depth and requires a second procedure.

- Step 2 (Redraping): The lower flap is undermined and secured at a lower height of tarsus. It addresses almost all of the ectropion. The second step should be considered to prevent further complications from secondary eyelid operations such as formation of triple folds and recurrent ectropion. The surgeon must take care not to allow a new adhesion from forming in the previous fold location. This adhesion can be prevented by the introduction of the orbital fat and septum into the space between the aponeurosis and the orbicularis muscle and by orbicularis muscle enforcement. If the deep fold remains persistent, a third step may be necessary.

- Step 3 (Tarsal scoring) (FIGURE 3-16): The lower flap is undermined until the eyelash follicles are exposed. The tarsal plate is scored at a 45-degree angle, just above the eyelash line. With this procedure, eyelash take on a more entropic orientation. This procedure is indicated for involutional ectropion, long-standing severe ectropion, and ectropion without stretched lower flap skin.

The important thing to consider in correction of ectropion is that a significant amount of ectropion that is visible on the operating table can be observed to have spontaneously resolved at a follow up visit. As such, complete removal of ectropion can eventually lead to shallow fold or entropion. Therefore, the operator must carefully decide the degree to which an ectropion is corrected.

Shallow or lost eyelid folds are corrected in a similar manner to neutral folds, by open blepharoplasty. Despite a complete loss of fold, however, the lower flap can still have severe adhesions on the lower flap and require adhesiolysis. If no such adhesions are present, the lower flap should have enough laxity to allow for adequate fixation at the desired height. It is important to note that patients with loss of fold usually have resistant eyelids, and the success of secondary operation is dependent on the surgeon's ability to deconstruct the elements from previous operation and quarantine such elements away from the newly created crease.

Failures after correction of high crease

Failure rates for high fold correction can be unacceptably high for surgeons who do

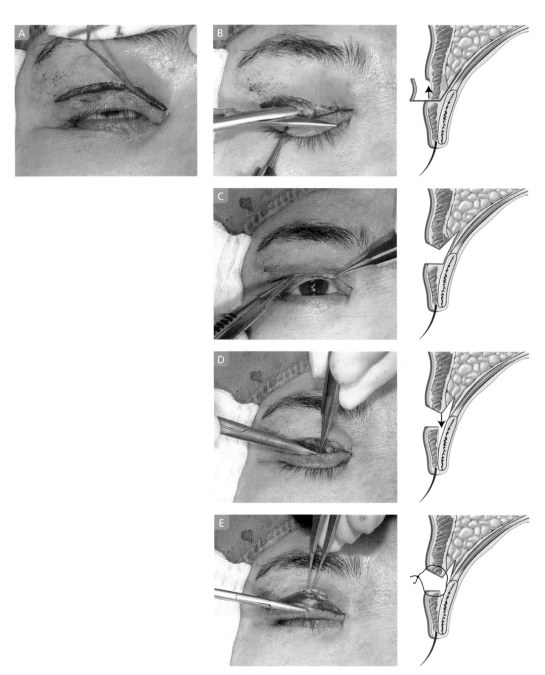

FIGURE 3-17 • Correction of high fold.
A. Excision of skin between pre-existing high crease and newly created low crease.
B. Dissection through the preaponeurotic layer.
C. Demonstration of eyelid excursion with the freely mobilized upper flap.
D. Any remaining ectropion can be resolved by mobilization of lower flap.
E. The lower flap is fixed at a lower point.

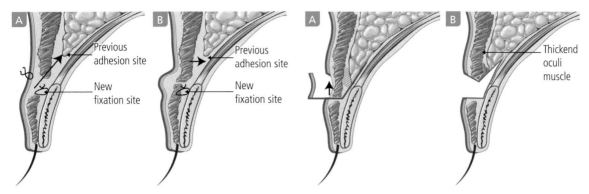

FIGURE 3-18 • Major complication after high fold correction. **A.** Ectropion results from incomplete lysis of adhesion. **B.** Triple fold results from re-adhesion.

FIGURE 3-19 • Skin excision. **A.** Skin excision and lysis of adhesion. **B.** Thickened oculi muscle.

not grasp the fundamental principle behind secondary operations – that unwanted adhesion is the enemy. The technical consequence is that surgeons do not completely release the tissue around the old eyelid crease. That is the primary reason for problems after high crease corrections. The secondary reason for failure is from re-adhesion of the tissue that was adequately freed. The two major problems that occur after high fold correction are ectropion and multiple folds **(FIGURE 3-18)**.

With incomplete lysis of adhesions or with re-adhesion, there is an ectropion of the upper eyelid with a crease that appears to be change height. With the eyes closed, the crease seems lowered as intended. However, the same crease does not appear lowered when the eyes are open because the skin is expanded and bunched from the everted eyelid.

Triple fold (multiple eyelid creases) can form after correction of high creases. In such post-secondary blepharoplasty patients, each crease represents the fixations performed in primary and secondary operation, where the lower crease is the desired crease and the higher crease had re-appeared at the sight of the initial operation. Even after complete adhesiolysis, the posterior lamella can re-adhere to the anterior lamella. The problem of triple folds is so common that it is discussed as its own topic in later part of this chapter.

To prevent these secondary complications, the surgeon must maintain sufficient tissue volume, thoroughly free the adhered tissue planes, and make efforts to prevent re-adhesion. To accomplish this, it is important to abide by the following guidelines.

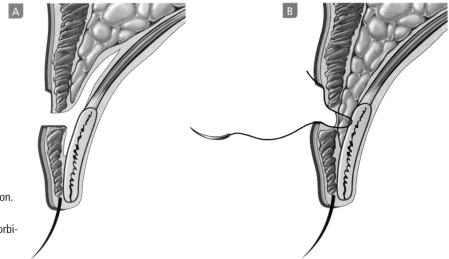

FIGURE 3-20 •
A. Pre-aponeurotic dissection.
B. Orbital fat interposition between aponeurosis and orbicularis muscle.

- Resect only the skin and leave the scar tissue to reinforce the upper flap **(FIGURE 3-17A, 3-19).**

- If the upper flap lacks sufficient soft tissue bulk, the orbital fat along with the septum can be lowered to add volume to the upper flap and also provide a gliding membrane between the orbicularis oculi and the levator aponeurosis. This latter function of interposition flap is extremely important in preventing re-adhesion of separated elements **(FIGURE 3-20).**

- In the same manner, the orbicularis muscle can be used as an interposition flap **(FIGURE 3-21).** Not only will it add volume to the area in risk of triple fold formation but also it has a great effect in not to meet the previous adhesion areas correcting or preventing triple folds.

- If there is insufficient orbital fat or orbicularis muscle, ROOF flap can be elevated for reinforcement. Dermofat graft, fat graft, or microfat injection deep to the orbicularis oculi can be alternative solutions and also effective in lowering the risk of re-adhesion.

- To increase the resistance to inward folding of skin at the initial operative site, a bulky roll of upper flap can be made by suturing the skin and orbicularis together after skin closure. The needle is passed through the skin and orbicularis oculi beneath the new crease, than through the orbicularis oculi and skin of the upper flap. In addition to increasing eyelid resistance along the length of old crease, it separates the anterior lamellar from the posterior lamella **(FIGURE 3-22).**

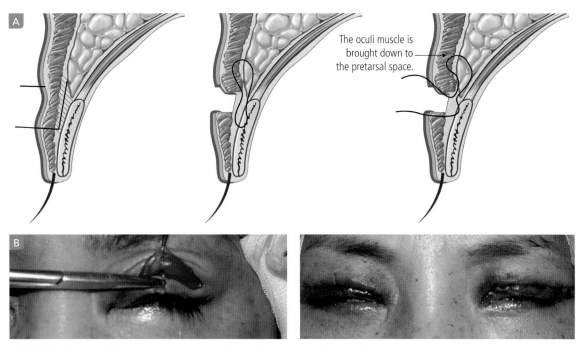

The oculi muscle is brought down to the pretarsal space.

FIGURE 3-21 • **A.** Orbicularis muscle interposition. **B.** Postoperative photograph.

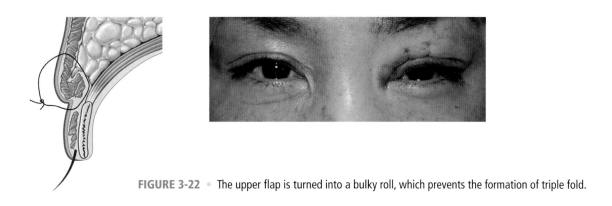

FIGURE 3-22 • The upper flap is turned into a bulky roll, which prevents the formation of triple fold.

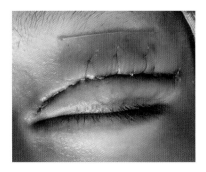

FIGURE 3-23 • Duoderm is used as a splint.

- Adhesive tape or duoderm can be used as a splint to increase fold-resistance in the immediate postoperative period **(FIGURE 3-23)**.
- If correction of eversion is made difficult due to severe adhesion, injection or spraying diluted steroids may help in the postoperative period.
- Excessive skin excision will result in the lower crease being pulled up towards the eyebrows, resulting in eversion. To prevent this, the lower flap can be fixed to the tarsal plate by securing it to a partial purchase in the tarsal plate during closure. This is effective in counteracting the upward pull from the taught eyelid skin **(FIGURE 3-17D, 3-22)**.
- Skin deficiency can be partially offset by undermining a 2-mm margin of skin in the upper flap.

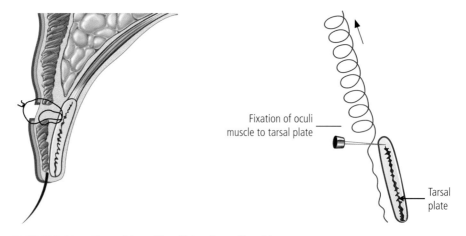

Fixation of oculi muscle to tarsal plate

Tarsal plate

FIGURE 3-24 • The problem of insufficient lower flap skin.
The lower flap should be fixated to the tarsal plate to prevent stretching of the skin by the levator mechanism.

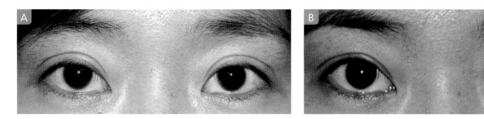

FIGURE 3-25 • Correction of high fold by lowering the crease.

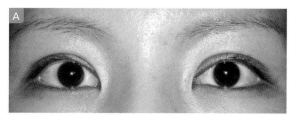
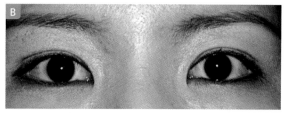

FIGURE 3-26 • Correction of high fold by lowering the fixation point.

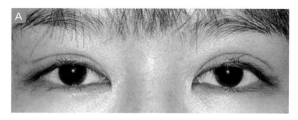
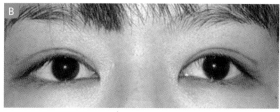

FIGURE 3-27 • Correction of high fold secondary to ptosis correction.

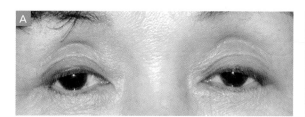
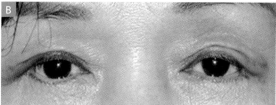

FIGURE 3-28 • Correction of high fold by crease mobilization and fat injection.

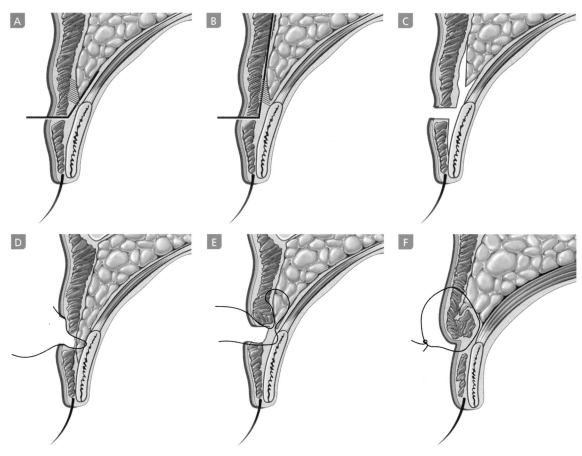

FIGURE 3-29 • **A.** Preaponeurotic layer dissection. **B.** Preseptal layer dissection. **C.** After preaponeurotic dissection and preseptal dissection. **D.** Orbital fat interposition. **E.** Orbicularis muscle pulling down. **F.** Skin & muscle roll.

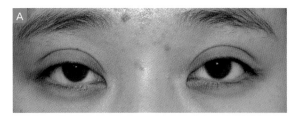

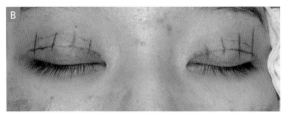

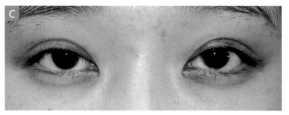

FIGURE 3-30 • High fold correction without skin excision.
A. Before surgery.
B. Upper line: pre-existing crease. Lower line: new crease design.
C. After surgery

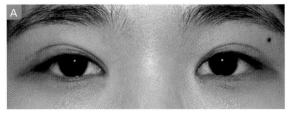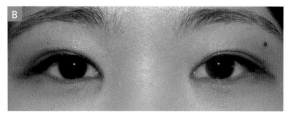

FIGURE 3-31 • High fold correction without skin excision.
A. Before surgery. **B.** After surgery.

PRETARSAL FULLNESS

Also called "sausage eyelid" among Korean patients, pretarsal fullness describes the unwanted soft tissue projection in the area over the tarsal plate in post-blepharoplasty eyelids. Commonly, pretarsal fullness is observed with high creases. Preoperative factors that predict pretarsal fullness include thick eyelid skin and orbicularis muscle. Patients with these features should receive eyelid folds which are designed lower than usual in order to counteract this propensity.

Pretarsal fullness increases in proportion to the square of the height of the pretarsal soft tissue compartment, which implies that small changes in height can result in great changes in volume of this compartment **(FIGURE 3-32)**. For example, an eyelid crease that changes height from 4 to 3 mm when opening the eye will have a volume reduction close to 50%(9/16). Another type of pretarsal fullness is caused by the abundance of pretarsal scar tissue.

Correction of pretarsal fullness

A common misconception is that pretarsal fullness can be corrected by removing the contents of this compartment such as the pretarsal portion of orbicularis muscle. This attempt at reducing volume is futile for several reasons. One, the removed volume is replaced with fibrous connective tissue. Two, this fibrous tissue interferes with the accordion effect of fold height being reduced with opening the eye. This decrease in elasticity results in static fullness of the compartment. Three, the actual volume represented in pretarsal fullness is the lowermost 2-4 mm of an

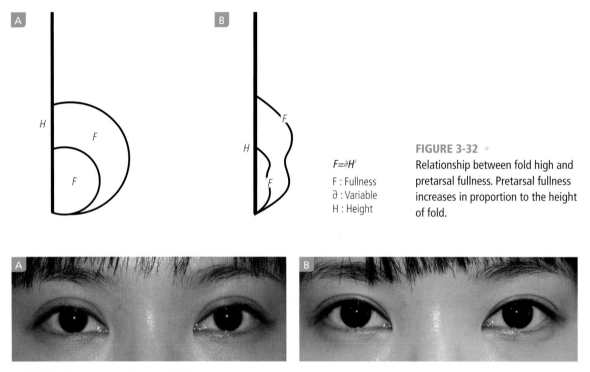

$F=∂H^2$

F : Fullness
∂ : Variable
H : Height

FIGURE 3-32 •

Relationship between fold high and pretarsal fullness. Pretarsal fullness increases in proportion to the height of fold.

FIGURE 3-33 • A case of pretarsal fullness.
A & B. Before and after corrective operation.

open eyelid from the ciliary margin. Removing soft tissue in this area is fraught with difficulty because of the eyelash follicles and the marginal arterial arcade.

To decrease the soft tissue volume in the pretarsal area, one must recognize the height-volume relationship mentioned above. Once this principle is understood, the technical solution is to perform a secondary operation (open blepharoplasty) to lower the crease and effectively reducing the height. The technical details for this were discussed in the previous section.

ASYMMETRY

From the perspective of clinical management, there are two main causes of postoperative eyelid asymmetry. Inexperienced surgeons often operated on a pre-existing asymmetry which was not noticed during the preoperative examination

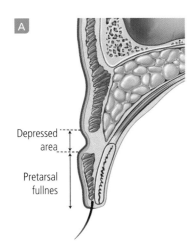
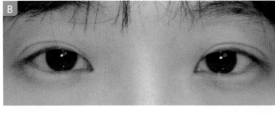
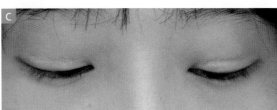

Depressed area

Pretarsal fullnes

FIGURE 3-34 •
A. Scar depression and pretarsal fullness. **B & C.** In this patient, excessive excision of oculi muscle has resulted in the depressed scar, which has resulted in para-doxical increase in pretarsal fullness.

and therefore was not discussed with the patient during the preoperative consultation. A thorough examination should include palpebral fissure height, redundancy of the eyelid skin, height of the brow, and unequal eyelashes.

A less common cause of eyelid asymmetry is technical failure on the part of the surgeon, whose operative maneuvers are not self-consistent from the left to the right eyelid. Slight variations in design, incision, soft tissue removal, and fixation can result in significant differences in overall outcome.

Preexisting asymmetry

Contributing factors for preexisting asymmetry include one-sided blepharoptosis, differences in eyelid laxity, brow height, crease height, and crease shape.

Patients are usually more sensitive about fold height than palpebral fissure height differences. Any existing blepharoptosis should be corrected before double eyelidplasty, but if the difference is minimal and the patient does not want a blepharoptosis operation, the new eyelid crease should be made lower in the ptotic eyelid.

Unequal skin redundancy should be addressed by a greater amount of skin excision, of course. While doing so, it is important to adjust the lower margin such that the crease height is equal on both eyelids. An attempt to correct asymmetry by varying the crease height is not recommended, since it is technically demanding. Even if the resulting crease height appears equal on primary gaze, there will be a difference upon downward or upward gaze. Additionally, downward gaze will

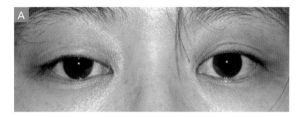
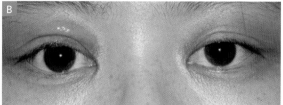

FIGURE 3-35 • Asymmetric crease height due to the asymmetry in underlying levator function. Before and after correction.

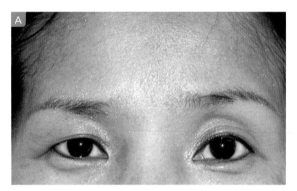
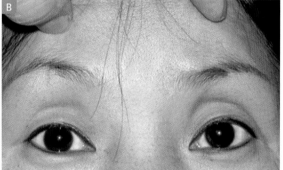

FIGURE 3-36 • **A.** In this patient, the asymmetry is due to asymmetry in brow ptosis. **B.** Manual elevation of the brows demonstrate that the eyelid creases themselves are in fact symmetric.

accentuate pretarsal fullness on the side with skin redundancy (FIGURE 3-35).

Correcting the brow asymmetry is the general rule. However, if the patient does not wish for an additional operation or if the asymmetry is not great enough to warrant the operation, the principle used for redundant skin applies as well. Excising skin on the side of elevated may be suboptimal, but it is extremely practical in clinical setting – provided that patients are counselled adequately regarding postoperative outcomes (FIGURE 3-36).

When both eyelid creases are higher than usual, the difference usually does not lead to noticeable asymmetry. In contrast, lower creases with asymmetric height will be extremely obvious. The palpebral fissure with lower fold, or no fold at all, will appear smaller because the skin looks weighed down (FIGURE 3-37). This situation is often overlooked or mistaken for asymmetric blepharoptosis. When asymmetry of this type is suspected, the palpebral fissure should be compared from left to right while using a bougie to create equal eyelid. The operation should be carried out in the usual manner - ignoring the illusion of asymmetry - by designing both folds at

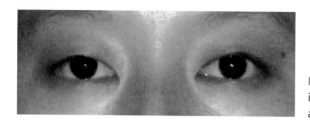

FIGURE 3-37 ● In the left eye, the inside fold is deep, which gives the appearance of a larger palpebral fissure.

the same height.

MULTIPLE CREASES (TRIPLE FOLDS)

Multiple eyelid creases, or triple folds, creases can form from various reasons and can be classified by clinical presentation.

Primary triple folds are formed in patients without any prior surgical history in patients experiencing the loss of fat volume (subcutaneous or deep fat) in the upper eyelid above a naturaly existing supratarsal fold. This presentation is within the spectrum of sunken eyelids and develops over a relatively longer time period in elderly patients and in patients who lose significant body weight.

Secondary triple folds are present in patients after the index blepharoplasty. Overzealous soft tissue removal in the upper flap can decrease fold-resistance of the eyelid and result in the extra eyelid crease above the surgically-created fold. The height of triple fold is different according to the over excision component of soft tissue. The height increases in the order of orbicularis muscle, retro-orbicularis oculi fat, and orbital fat (FIGURE 3-38). In particular, removal of retro-orbicularis oculi fat (ROOF) in the medial eyelid may lead to triple fold and should be avoided. At times, pretarsal or the preaponeurotic soft tissue is removed to facilitate adhesion and formation of eyelid crease. However, removal of this tissue above the point of fixation should be avoided because doing so may result in triple fold formation (FIGURE 3-39, 3-40).

Tertiary triple folds form after secondary operations for correction of high fold, ectropion, or eyelid retraction. The extra creases are all consequences of re-adhesion of the deconstructed fold (FIGURE 3-41).

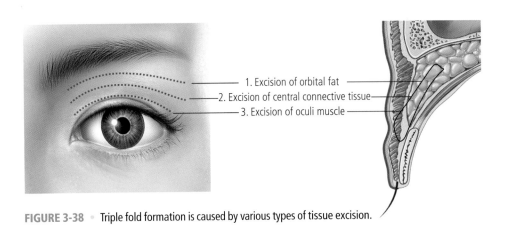

1. Excision of orbital fat
2. Excision of central connective tissue
3. Excision of oculi muscle

FIGURE 3-38 • Triple fold formation is caused by various types of tissue excision.

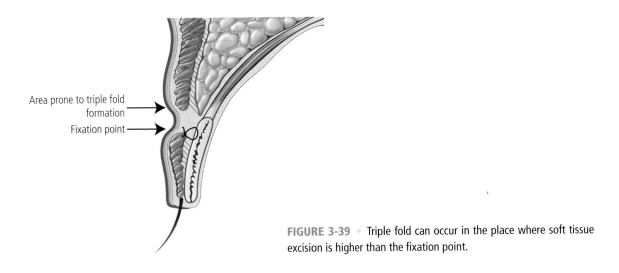

Area prone to triple fold formation

Fixation point

FIGURE 3-39 • Triple fold can occur in the place where soft tissue excision is higher than the fixation point.

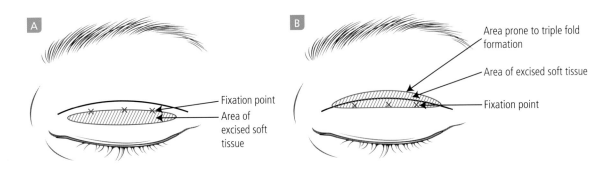

Fixation point
Area of excised soft tissue

Area prone to triple fold formation
Area of excised soft tissue
Fixation point

FIGURE 3-40 • If soft tissue is excised above the fixation point, triple fold formation is possible.
A. The fixation points should be made at the upper most portion of tissue excision. **B.** Soft tissue excision above the fixation point can lead to additional crease.

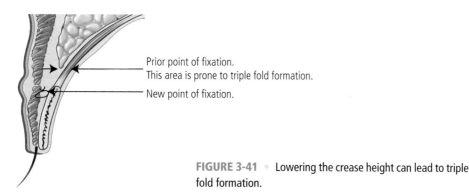

Prior point of fixation.
This area is prone to triple fold formation.
New point of fixation.

FIGURE 3-41 • Lowering the crease height can lead to triple fold formation.

Correction

If the extraneous crease is shallow, fat injection alone might be enough to bolster the skin and prevent further progression of the crease. It required open access is required for meticulous release of adhesions and to perform preventive measures.

The upper flap should be released between the levator aponeurosis and orbital septum. Usually, this is sufficient in itself in releasing the adhesion forming the extraneous crease. If not, the space between postorbicularis fascia and the orbital septum should be cleared for additional separation of outer and inner elements. The later plane of dissection should be more extensive and extend superiorly. Re-adhesion is prevented by inferior displacement of well-organized septum and orbital fat between the orbicularis oculi and the levator muscle. The postorbicularis fascia and muscle is lowered from previous site of adhesion and anchored to the tarsal plate (**FIGURE 3-38**).

Another method to prevent readhesion is to create a roll with the skin and orbicularis oculi muscle of the upper flap. The method is to pass the needle under-through the skin and orbicularis oculi just beneath the crease, then through the orbicularis oculi and skin of the upper flap creating a slightly bunched kind of roll (**FIGURE 3-39**). Applying adhesive tape to an area in high risk of triple fold can also be effective (**FIGURE 3-40**).

Blepharoptosis often coexists with multiple creases and contributes to the formation of the extraneous crease. As such, all such ptosis should be corrected simultaneously at the time of triple fold correction.

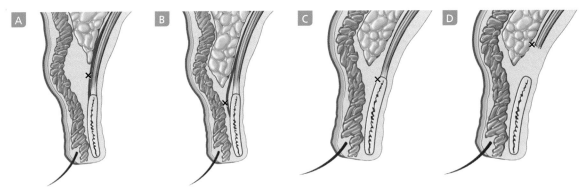

FIGURE 3-42 • **A.** Prior to ptosis correction. **B.** After ptosis correction, the prior point of eyelid crease (marked 'X') is prone to triple fold formation. **C.** Prior to correction of retraction. **D.** After correction of retraction, the prior point of eyelid crease (marked 'X') is prone to triple fold formation at a higher location.

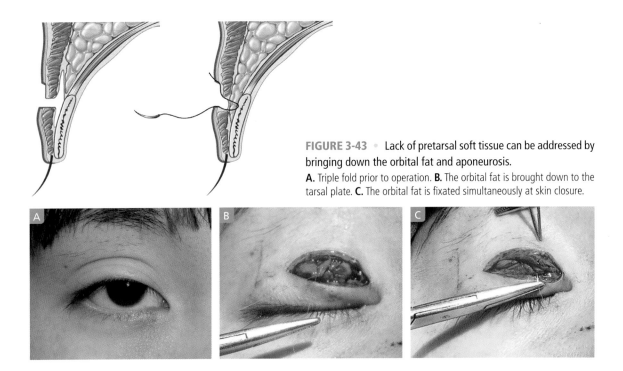

FIGURE 3-43 • Lack of pretarsal soft tissue can be addressed by bringing down the orbital fat and aponeurosis.
A. Triple fold prior to operation. **B.** The orbital fat is brought down to the tarsal plate. **C.** The orbital fat is fixated simultaneously at skin closure.

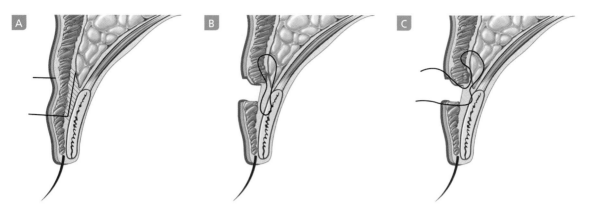

FIGURE 3-44 • Prevention or correction of triple fold formation.
A. Preaponeurotic dissection. **B.** Oculi muscle and orbital fat interposition. **C.** Oculi muscle and orbital fat interposition during skin suture.

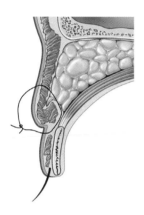

FIGURE 3-45 • Prevention or correction of triple fold formation.
Skin and oculi muscle roll.

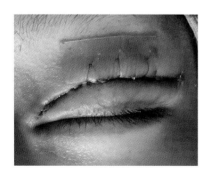

FIGURE 3-46 • Duoderm is used to splint the area prone to triple fold formation.

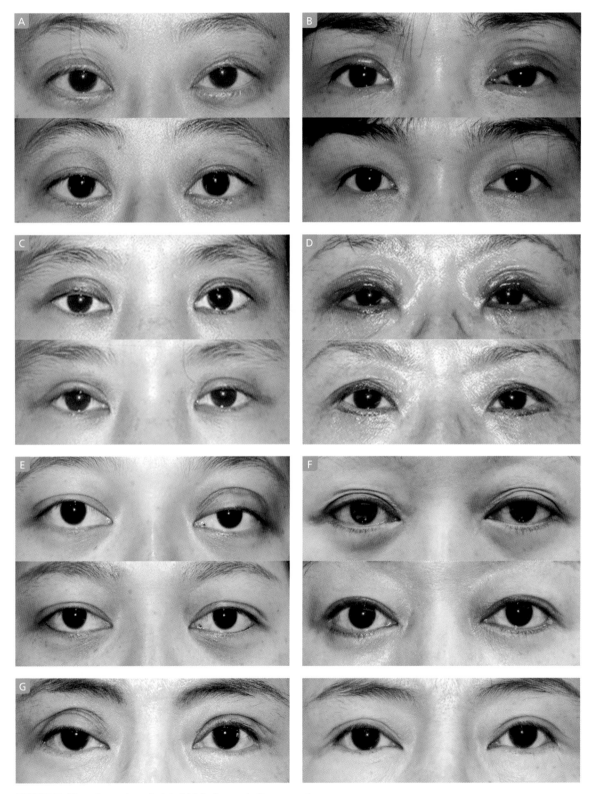

FIGURE 3-47 • Correction of triple fold (before and after surgery).

SUNKEN EYELID/PRIMARY TRIPLE FOLD

Sunken eyelids occur from deficiency of orbital fat or soft tissue and rarely from adhesion between superficial and deep structures. For this reason, primary triple fold and sunken eyelids can be thought of as a single clinical entity. As such, treatment for sunken eyelid is similar to treatments for primary triple fold.

Correction

The lost volume of soft tissue can be replenished by fat injection, dermofat graft, or grafting of other soft tissues such as muscle fascia **(FIGURE 3-48)**.

Fat injection to the subcutaneous layer or oculi muscle layer can create irregularity in texture. Microfat injection in the deeper plane between orbicularis oculi muscle and septum (RROF) reduces the potential for surface irregularity. However, injecting into the deeper layer has the potential for levator muscle injury, which would result in mechanical blepharoptosis. Injection into the retroorbicularis oculi fat (ROOF) can also cause belpharoptosis from the added weight. However, this is usually transient. Nevertheless, the risk of this complication can be minimized by injecting the fat just above the periosteum while the upper eyelid is pulled upward and the eyes wide open. This will ensure that the levator muscle is well within the orbital rim and decrease the weight burden on the muscle **(FIGURE 3-49)**.

Injecting fat into the orbicularis oculi muscle can be effective for a triple fold caused by a adhesion within a superficial layer. In most cases, however, this should be meticulously done because of the problem with surface irregularities.

Fat can be injected beneath the orbital septum if the septum can be visualized by an incision. Graft survival rate is relatively high with minimal risk for surface irregularity or lump formation with closed eyelids. It is however not a widely practiced technique and may represent a challenge in technical knowhow.

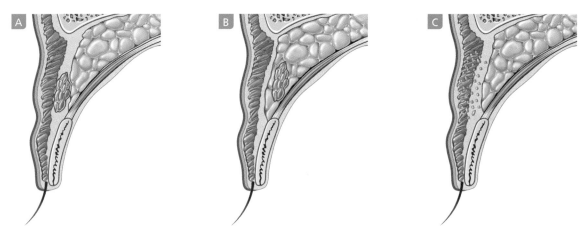

FIGURE 3-48 • Fat graft for sunken eyelid.
A. Preseptal fat graft. **B.** Retroseptal fat graft. **C.** Fat injection on retro-orbicularis oculi layer.

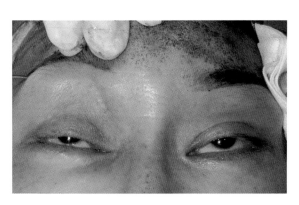

FIGURE 3-49 • Fat injection into the ROOF.
The fat graft should be injected while the levator muscle is retracted (open eyelid) and the eyebrows are retracted. This minimizes the risk of intramuscular injection of the fat graft.

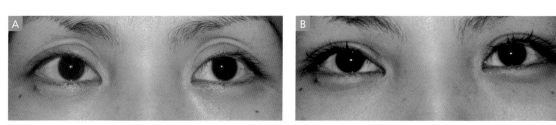

FIGURE 3-50 • Fat injection for correction of sunken eyelid.

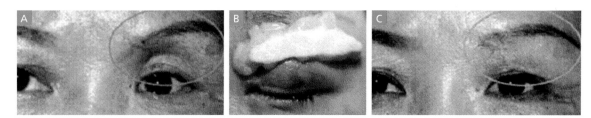

FIGURE 3-51 • Dermofat graft for correction of sunken eyelid.

BLEPHAROPTOSIS

In the immediate postoperative period, mild-to-moderate blepharoptosis may simply be due to edema or local anesthesia effect, which is transient and will disappear with the edema. If a moderate-to-severe blepharoptosis does not recede with edema, however, the surgeon must suspect the possibility of injury to the levator mechanism **(FIGURE 3-52)**.

The most common location at which the levator mechanism is violated is at the junction between levator aponeurosis and the upper border of tarsal plate. While soft tissue excision along the top margin of tarsal plate is necessary at times to induce orbicularis muscle-tarsal fixation, removal of soft tissue superior to tarsal plate can violate the fibers connecting the aponeurosis to the plate. The resulting blepharoptosis may not be noticed in the immediate postoperative period because of the edema and because of the compensation of Muller muscle. Over the next several years, the Muller muscle is undergoes mechanical failure from the demand of opening the eyelid without the help of levator aponeurosis. This is the most likely scenario for delayed blepharoptosis in patients who has had double eyelid operations more than a decade ago.

The levator function can be tested by elevating the ptotic eyelid skin and is especially important for elderly patients. Compensating brow elevation may also mask minor blepharoptosis. As stated above, minor unilateral blepharoptosis can easily be missed and become a cause for unexpected postoperative asymmetry. Likewise,

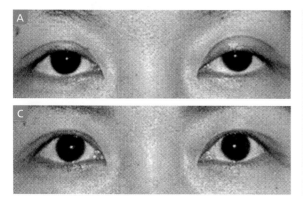
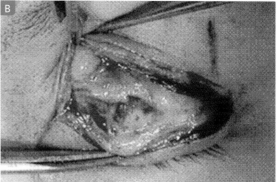

FIGURE 3-52 • Bilateral post-traumatic ptosis.
A. Preoperative photograph. **B.** Intraoperative examination reveals disinsertion of levator muscle. **C.** Postoperative photograph.

it is important to distinguish between true ptosis (levator failure) and dermatochalasis (drooping skin) in the elderly patients.

If levator muscle injury is recognized, the surgeon should consider which tissue to advance and by how much. This advancement would stretch out the levator or the Muller muscle, so it is important to assess the tension through the full thickness of levator mechanism. Lacerations should be approximated and plicated minimally so that the Muller muscle is minimally stretched. In the injury was to the upper septum with resultant adhesion, simply releasing the adhesion may free the levator and correct the blepharoptosis (FIGURE 3-53).

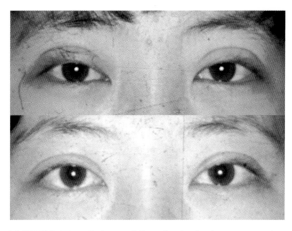

FIGURE 3-53 • Release of the adhesion in the upper portion of aponeurosis has allowed the eyelid to retract to the neutral position.

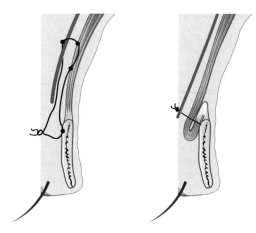

FIGURE 3-54 • Müller plication and levator advancement for correction of ptosis.
Purple: levator aponeurosis. Red: Müller muscle.

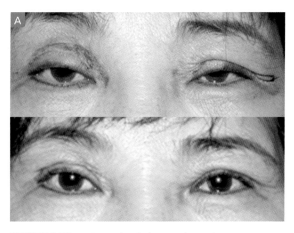

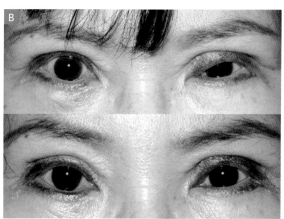

FIGURE 3-55 • Correction in iatrogenic ptosis.

In iatrogenic blepharoptosis cases, the patient must understand beforehand the goals and limitations of the operation. The goal is to achieve normal and symmetric field of vision on primary gaze. However, the levator muscle may lack the normal range of motion from fibrotic changes, and the patient must understand that lid lag or lagophthalmos can persist afterwards.

REMOVAL OF THE EYELID FOLD

Several facts must be presented by the surgeon and those facts understood by the patient before an operation is carried out to remove a surgically created eyelid fold. The first fact is that a visible scar will be present even when the eyes are open. The second is that the fold can reappear with time. The third is that the eyelid may

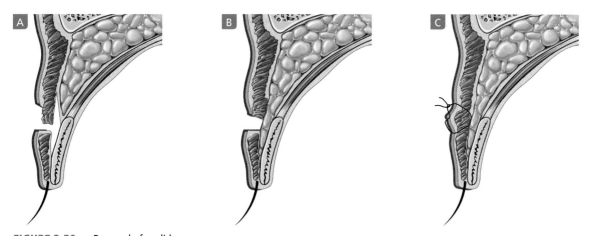

FIGURE 3-56 • Removal of eyelid crease.
A. Removal of scar tissue. **B.** Lysis of adhesion and interposition of orbital fat. **C.** Vertical mattress suture of skin and oculi muscle.

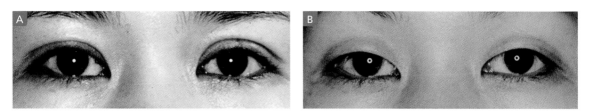

FIGURE 3-57 • Before and after removal of the eyelid creases.

appear and feel bulkier due to the scar tissue, injection of fat graft, or inferior displacement of fat and septum down to the area in risk of re-adhesion.

Because of these potential issues, the author usually recommends an inner eyelid fold rather than total removal of eyelid fold. Inner eyelid folds are created in a similar manner to the operation correcting high creases. The adhesion forming the existing crease is deconstructed, and orbital fat and septum is interposed between the layers to prevent re-adhesion. Eversion should be achieved during skin closure. The incision site is taped for longer than usual 3-5 days.

CONCLUSION

The complications that arise after primary and secondary blepharoplasty operations are too numerous to allow a comprehensive discussion within a chapter. However, the basic principles of reconstructive surgery are applicable to a majority of these complications. The first principle is to understand the normal and abnormal function and anatomy – in this case those of the eyelid. The second principle is to undo, or deconstruct the postoperative tissue changes causing the complication. The third principle is to re-do the initial operation without making the same mistake.

Surgical outcomes are beautiful because the underlying principle orchestrating the surgeon through the operation is beautiful.

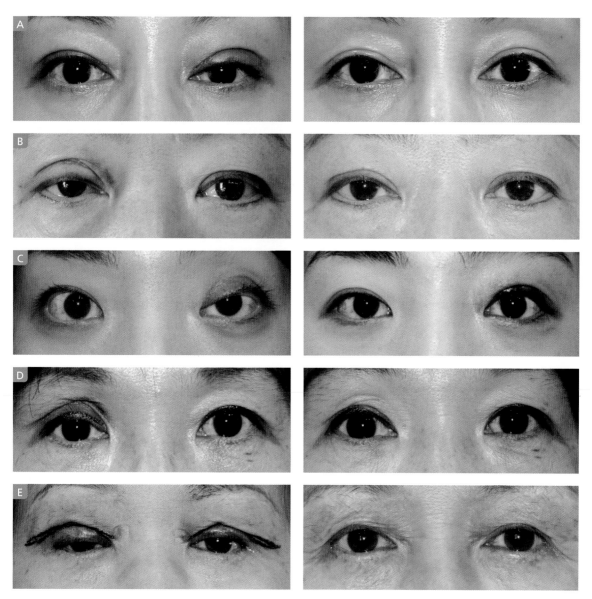

FIGURE 3-58 • Early correction of unfavorable operative outcomes.
Left: Preoperative photographs. Right: Postoperative photographs.

REFERENCES

1. Kim YW, Park HJ, Kim S : Secondary Correction of Unsatisfactory Blepharoplasty: Removing Multilaminated Septal Structures and Grafting of Preaponeurotic Fat. Plast Reconstr Surg 106:1399, 2000.
2. Chen WP : The Concept of a Glide Zone as It Relates to Upper Lid Crease, Lid Fold, and Application in Upper Blepharoplasty. Plast Reconstr Surg 119:379, 2007.
3. Kim YW, Park HJ, Kim S : Revision of Unfavorable Double Eyelid Operation by Repositioning of Preaponeurotic Fat. J Korean Soc Plast Reconstr Surg 27:99, 2000.

EPICANTHOPLASTY

- Surgical indication
- Surgical technique
- Revision epicanthoplasty

Epicanthal folds can give off the appearance of blunted affect in patients. The medial borders of palpebral fissure are farther apart (increased interepicanthal distance), and this tends to create the illusion of hypertelorism. The folds decrease the horizontal length of palpebral fissure. The rotund shape of medial palpebral border is undesirable in a wide array of aesthetic contexts.

SURGICAL INDICATION

1. Desire for a more alert appearance with lengthening horizontal palpebral fissure
2. Above average intercanthal distance
3. The presence of epicanthal fold

The following factors are important for determining the type and extent of epicanthoplasty appropriate for each patient:

1. Lacrimal caruncle exposure
2. Intercanthal distance
3. Shape and color of the lacrimal caruncle

The medial palpebral fissure

The medial palpebral fissure is accentuated by the mucosal flesh consisting of lacrimal caruncle and semilunaris. The degree to which this mucosal surface is exposed varies significantly across patients. A closed or covered medial fissure is associated with a blunted or inattentive appearance (FIGURE 4-1), whereas a widely open medial fissure can be mistaken for an aggressive stare. In patients without significant epicanthal fold, approximately one-third of this mucosal surface is covered. This is a relatively good starting point for what constitutes an attractive media palpebral fissure.

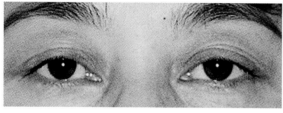 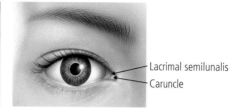

Lacrimal semilunalis
Caruncle

FIGURE 4-1 • A patient with congenitally overexposed lacrimal caruncle.

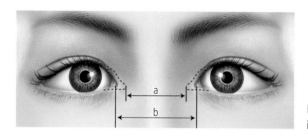

FIGURE 4-2 • The difference in intercanthal distance (a) and interepicanthal distance (b).

Intercanthal and interepicanthal distances

Epicanthoplasty is an operation designed to decrease the interepicanthal distance and does not have any effect on the intercanthal distance (**FIGURE 4-2**).

Interepicanthal distance exists in harmony with horizontal features of the face, such as palpebral fissure and the full width of midface. The mean interepicanthal width is around 35 mm in the Korean population, though the recent trend has been for decreasing width. A width less than 30 mm may be too narrow even for patients with hypotelorism.

Other factors influencing epicanthoplasty

Epicanthoplasty should be conservative for several reasons. A larger proportion of the mucosa should be left covered, if the mucosal surface is too erythematous or shaded or if the medial palpebral fissure assumes the shape of a hook (**FIGURE 4-3**).

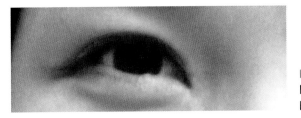

FIGURE 4-3 • If retraction of the epicanthal fold reveals a hook-shaped medial canthus underneath, the fold should not be opened too widely.

SURGICAL TECHNIQUE

Among various methods, the ideal epicanthoplasty observes three conditions:

1. Minimal scarring

2. Removal of epicanthal fold

3. Natural shape of the medial palpebral fissure

Postoperative scarring is minimized by the following:

1. The smallest incision possible

2. Inconspicuous site of incision

3. Minimal number of skin flaps, if such flaps are necessary

Oh method of skin redraping

The skin draping method by Oh et al. utilizes a pericilliary incision and therefore conceals the postoperative scar within a naturally occurring facial line. The fibrous connective tissue between the orbicularis muscle and skin is responsible for the banding effect of the epicanthal fold. The merit behind this technique is that this fibrous tissue is released, while the skin is redraped. Division of the fibrous tissue does not require a large access, and therefore, the incisions tend to be smaller with this technique.

Surgical technique

Design (FIGURE 4-5A)

The incision begins with a gentle traction of the epicanthal fold. The midpoint of

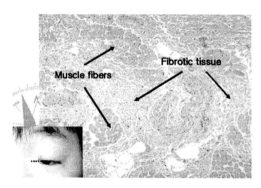

FIGURE 4-4 • Connective tissue in a cross section of epicanthal fold. Fibrous tissue can be found from just deep to dermis down to the orbicularis muscle layer.
(Source: J.W.Park)

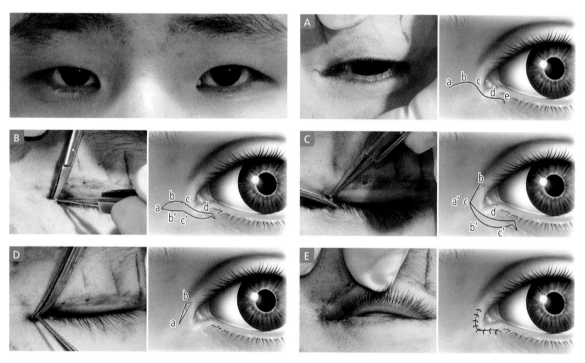

FIGURE 4-5 • Operative details for epicanthoplasty.

incision, 'c', is marked at the inner skin over the medial canthus. The epicanthal fold is allowed to relax, and the medial end of the incision, 'a', is marked over the skin directly anterior to point 'c'. The distance between 'a' and 'c' defines the magnitude of epicanthoplasty. Generally, these points should be distanced adequately to allow for tension free closure at the end of operation. Closure of the surgical wound with less than adequate tissue mobilization will promote hypertrophic response and lead to over-exposure of the lacrimal caruncle. The incision design is curved and incorporates point 'b' in the design, such that the lower skin flap has more material to be rotated laterally.

From point 'c', the design extends laterally along the pericilliary line of lower eyelid. This should not be too close to the upper margin and should be designed with a 2-3 mm offset. This lateral portion of the incision design should have a back cut that is approximately 110 degrees from the horizontal line. Curve 'c-d-e' becomes proportionally longer, as the epicanthal fold is opened wider.

Mobilization (FIGURE 4-5B)

The incision is carried through the dermis. The lower skin flap can be elevated along the subcutaneously, but the dissection plane that partially incorporates the orbicularis muscle fibers can be preferable to minimize tissue injury. This dissection must be performed in a diligent manner that protects the lacrimal canaliculus, which travels medially for 2 mm before inferomedially for 7 mm into the nasal cavity. In this technique, the incision is placed 2 mm inferior to the mucocutaneous junction. The lacrimal duct is relatively shallow, and the skin flap should be dissected with spreading instruments rather than with sharp instruments. Once the flap is sufficiently elevated, the epicanthal fold is released by dissecting the fibrous connective tissue (FIGURE 4-4).

Closure (FIGURE 4-5C)

The lower flap rotated such that point 'a' is sutured to point 'c' – effectively redraping the epicanthal skin. The lower wound margin will be longer than the upper margin, and this discrepancy should be divided evenly along the whole length of incision skin. If this accordion method does not resolve all of the length discrepancy, the remaining dog ear is resected and closed with a back cut.

Upper eyelid (FIGURE 4-5D)

Any dog-ear in the upper eyelid can be easily managed by a 2-3 mm excision of the excess skin.

Complications of this technique

1. Undercorrection and overcorrection
2. Medial pretarsal flatness or depression (FIGURE 4-6)

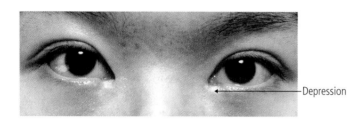

Depression

FIGURE 4-6 • An example of excessively exposed lacrimal mucosa.

In this patient, the exposure is not only in the horizontal but also in the vertical dimension. The deficiency of tissue in the medial portion of the lower eyelid margin has resulted in slope deformity of the medial corners.

3. Hyperpigmentation

4. Scarring

5. Skin lump at the ends of incision

6. Retraction or scleral show

In most cases, the medial palpebral fissure is opened adequately if there is no undue tension and skin redundancy at the time of suturing points 'a' to point 'c'. Overcorrection can be avoided by starting out with a smaller than expected incision and to extend this incision in minute increments while evaluating the tension in the skin flap.

One of the most difficult complications to manage is the exposure of inferior portion of the lacrimal caruncle. This is caused by excessive vertical skin tension during suture.

To avoid vertical exposure of lacrimal mucosa:

1. Vertical tension can be decreased by a larger inferior skin flap, which is accomplished by increasing the curvature of the line 'a-c' (**FIGURE 4-5A**). Slight excess in the lower flap is usually not a problem, except for patients with epiblepharon or entropion.

2. The incision should be 2-to-3 mm offset from the lower eyelid margin to decrease the vertical tension and, subsequently, to prevent vertical exposure of the lacrimal mucosa.

3. Point 'd' is the most likely to become depressed. In this area, the orbicularis muscle should not be elevated, and the skin dissection should stay superficial.

The risk of hypo/hyperpigmentation can be minimized by:

1. Dissection along the intramuscular plane and

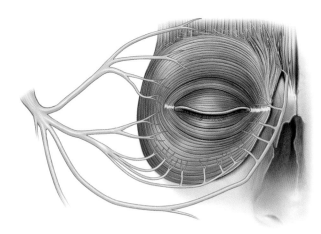

FIGURE 4-7 • The buccal branch of the facial nerve travels medially to medial canthus.

2. Avoiding hematoma and hemosiderin-related pigmentation.

The author prefers intramuscular dissection over subcutaneous dissection. The skin is extremely thin and adheres to the orbicularis muscle with dense fibrous connections. As such, the skin can be injured too easily with subcutaneous dissection.

A distal buccal branch of the facial nerve traverses next to the medial canthal tendon. This branch can be damaged, if the skin incision incorporates too much orbicularis muscle or if the muscle is excised **(FIGURE 4-7)**. The resulting nerve injury can lead to a mild degree of nocturnal lagophthalmos, and the operation most commonly associated with this complication is dacryocystorhinostomy. Fortunately, this type lagophthalmos usually resolves within 3 months. Excessive excision of the orbicularis muscle can also result in drooping of the lower eyelid and scleral show. This is most likely due to separation of the orbicularis muscle from the origin with resultant decrease in muscle tonicity.

It is important to protect the lacrimal duct when dissecting the lower eyelid flap. From the punctum, the lacrimal duct travels inferiorly for 2 mm, where it takes a medial course towards the nasal cavity. This initial vertical portion is very superficial and dives deeper after the medial turn. As such, the flap dissection must be superficial around the base of lacrimal punctum **(FIGURE 4-8)**.

Application

This technique can be applied in following situations:

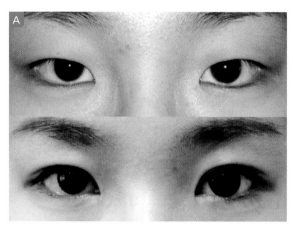
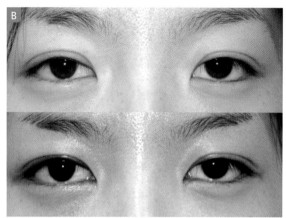

FIGURE 4-8 • Photographs before and after epicanthoplasty.

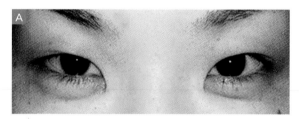
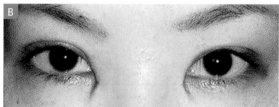

FIGURE 4-9 • In this patient, a combination of blepharoplasty and epicanthoplasty has produced a wider palpebral fissure but with a more pronounced epicanthal fold.

Epicanthal folds with adequately visible lacrimal mucosa

Generally, epicanthoplasty is defined by the elimination of the epicanthal fold and a simultaneous exposure of the lacrimal mucosa. At times, however, patients may present with epicanthal folds that do not obstruct the view of mucosa. In such cases (**FIGURE 4-9**), Oh epicanthoplasty should be modified in two ways. The medial portion of the incision should be shortened, and the fibrous tissue should be released nasally, inferiorly, and superiorly (**FIGURE 4-10, 4-11**). Otherwise, the fold can be released during a revision epicanthoplasty design (**FIGURE 4-11C**).

Epicanthal folds with lower eyelid entropion (**FIGURE 4-12, 4-13**)

Occasionally, epicanthal folds are accompanied by entropion, which is limited to the medial portion of the lower eyelid margin.

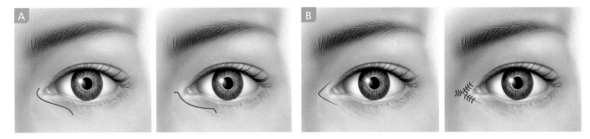

FIGURE 4-10 • Epicanthoplasty with minimal mucosal show.
A. The medial portion of incision can be extended superiorly or shortened. **B.** Prominent epicanthal folds can be addressed with a V-Y advancement flap.

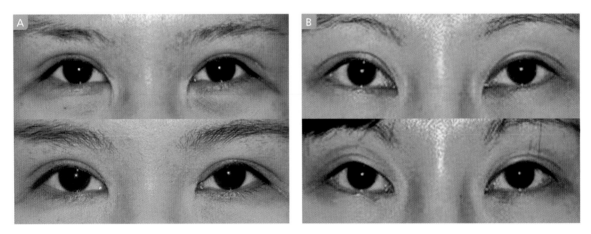

FIGURE 4-11 • Pre/postoperative photographs.
A. Removal of epicanthal fold without mucosal exposure. **B.** The epicanthal fold can be released during an revision epicanthoplasty design.

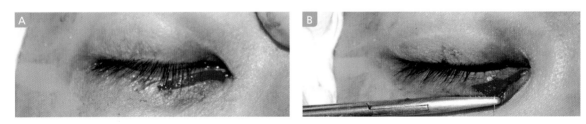

FIGURE 4-12 • Epicanthal fold with lower eyelid entropion.
A. The skin incision is extended along the portion of lower eyelid with entropion. **B.** The orbicularis muscle in the upper flap is fixed to the tarsal plate.

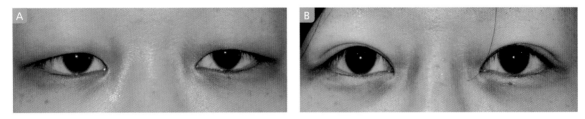

FIGURE 4-13 • Pre/postoperative photographs for correction of entropion via epicanthoplasty.

Surgical technique

If the epicanthal coexists with lower eyelid entropion, the subcilliary incision can be extended laterally. Correction of entropion will be addressed briefly, as it is discussed extensively in Chapter 6.

- There are no eyelashes from the inner canthal corner to the lacrimal punctum. As such, this portion of the lower eyelid incorporates the design described above.
- Lateral to the punctum, the incision is carried with a 2-mm offset from the eyelashes.
- The dissection is carried through the orbicularis muscle, and the tarsal plate is exposed.
- Orbicularis oculi muscle of the upper flap is fixed to the lower border of tarsus to create ectropion.
- The skin is closed.

The orbicularis muscle should not be excised to prevent loss of the pretarsal fullness.

Hiraga method of epicanthoplasty (FIGURE 4-14, 4-15)

Indication

1. The epicanthal fold itself is not prominent, but the view of lacrimal mucosa is obstructed mildly.
2. Post-epicanthoplasty patient who wishes for a secondary operation to widen the medial portion of fissure a little more.

In most situations, Oh epicanthoplasty can allow significant mobilization of soft tissue with minimally visible scar. For patients who wish for a less drastic change, Hiraga's method may be a simpler alternative with just as minimal of a postoperative scar. In this technique, a horizontal incision is made across the epicanthal fold, as much as needed for tensionless advancement. The incision is closed by bringing the to end points together, and the resulting dog-ears are excised.

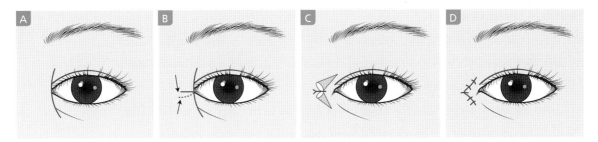

FIGURE 4-14 • Hiraga's method.
A. Preoperative state of the epicanthal fold. **B.** The length of horizontal incision is dependent on the amount of tissue to be advanced. **C.** The ending points of incision are brought together. Resulting dog-ears are excised. **D.** Postoperative state.

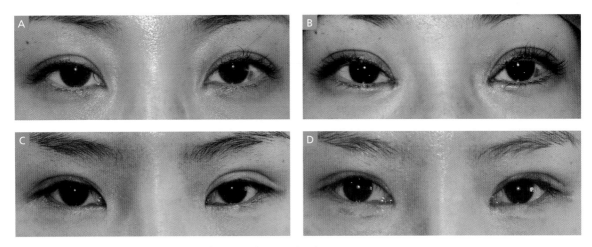

FIGURE 4-15 • Photographs before and after Hiraga's epicanthoplasty.
This simple technique is appropriate for patients without prominent epicanthal fold, who wish for more open medial fissures.

FREQUENTLY ASKED QUESTIONS

Q DOES EPICANTHOPLASTY WIDEN THE VERTICAL DIMENSIONS OF PALPEBRAL FISSURE?

A   The simple answer is 'yes'. The epicanthal band contributes a significant vertical force on the eyelids. The operation releases this band, and the resulting change in vertical vector will lead to a proportional increase in fissure height. The degree to which epicanthoplasty will change fissure height can be evaluated in the preoperative setting by manually eliminating this tension while the patient assumes a neutral gaze. Complete dissection of this band from the surrounding tissue should be avoided, as this may lead to scleral show.

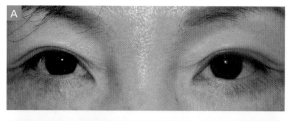
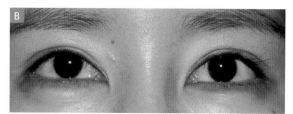
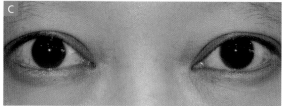

FIGURE 4-16 • Lacrimal mucosal exposure since birth.

REVISION EPICANTHOPLASTY

Epicanthal fold reconstruction is indicated in those patients with excessive exposure of the lacrimal mucosa. Such cases of excessive exposure of mucosa are caused most commonly by prior epicanthoplasty and less commonly by trauma or congenital etiology (FIGURE 4-16).

In the management of excessive exposure of lacrimal mucosa, the focus is directed at the horizontal aspect of the exposure. Medial pretarsal flatness or slope deformity is another serious problem after epicanthoplasty (FIGURE 4-6). In such cases, epicanthal folds should be reconstructed with elevation of the lower lid skin.

Operative method I) V-Y advancement with back-cut

(FIGURE 4-17)

1. The operative design assumes that the end of epicanthal fold, point 'd', will take place at the end point of the back cut.
2. A horizontal V-shaped incision is made over the epicanthal fold. The first design can be considered as a V-Y advancement. The W-shaped incision is used to minimize the length of postoperative scar.
3. The extent to which the lacrimal mucosa is covered by the epicanthal fold is determined by the degree of V-Y advancement. The subcutaneous layer is closed with 7-0 PDS suture, and this suture incorporates the deeper floor to eliminate

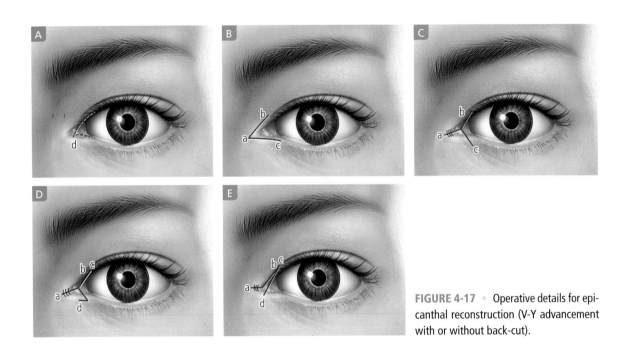

FIGURE 4-17 • Operative details for epicanthal reconstruction (V-Y advancement with or without back-cut).

any dead space.

4. From point 'c', a back-cut is extended at 45 degree. The end point of the back-cut, point 'd', will become the new end of the reconstructed epicanthal fold. An obtuse back-cut angle will pull down on the upper eyelid and result in a more prominent epicanthal fold. Conversely, a more acute back-cut angle will not effect eyelid positions as much, with a less prominent fold.

5. A Z-plasty is performed between the two flaps, with the lower back-cut flap transposed into the upper eyelid margin.

Operative method II) V-Y advancement (FIGURE 4-18)

1. V-shaped incision along the previous scar line
2. The V-Y advancement is secured using subcutaneous suture.
3. The triangular flap is excised partially.
4. Skin is closed.

In this method of epicanthal reconstruction, two important points to consider are the mobilization and shape of the epicanthal fold. The extent of mobilization

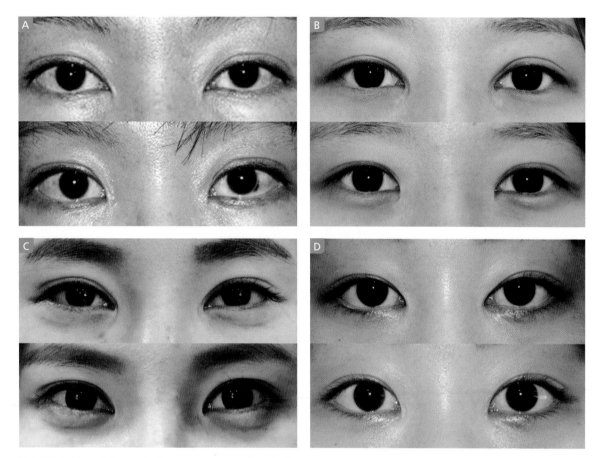

FIGURE 4-18 • Before and after reconstructive epicanthoplasty.
After epicanthal reconstruction, the lacrimal mucosa are less exposed. The increased interepicanthal distance has an effect of softening the "aggressive" appearance. Medial pretarsal flatness or slope deformity has resolved.

is determined at the time of V-Y advancement, by which the operator can approximate the extent to which the lacrimal mucosa is covered. The length of back-cut influences both the mobilization and shape of the fold. A shorter back-cut tends to make for a more obtuse medial canthus, whereas a longer back-cut will leave a greater portion of the lacrimal gland exposed.

Another consideration is scar visibility. Scar depression is the most significant contributing factor to conspicuousness of a scar. To decrease the risk of scar depression, the V-Y advancement should be closed with an underlying layer of subcutaneous sutures to decrease the tension and to use vertical mattress sutures to evert the wound margin.

Special cases of epicanthal reconstruction

Epicanthal fold removal with revision epicanthoplasty

The general understanding is that removal of epicanthal fold leads to exposure of the lacrimal mucosa. However, patients sometimes present with a widely exposed lacrimal mucosa, which is accompanied by prominent folds. In such cases, the epicanthal band can be transected at the time of subcutaneous dissection, after which the skin flaps are repositioned in Z-plasty (FIGURES 4-18 and 4-20).

Depressed scar after epicanthoplasty

Usually, epicanthoplasty is designed as close as possible to the lid margin. In the presence of severely depressed scar, however, the horizontal V-shaped incision is made along the depression to mobilize the depressed scar into the invisible area behind the fold. This results in a conversion of the out-fold upper eyelid crease into an in-fold one.

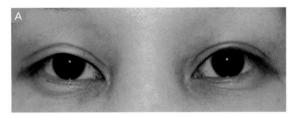 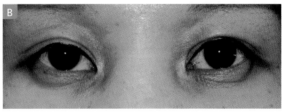

FIGURE 4-19 • Reconstructive epicanthoplasty in this patient has coverted the out-fold into an in-fold.

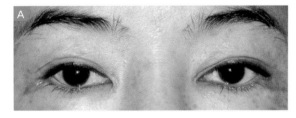 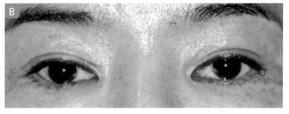

FIGURE 4-20 • In this patient, the epicanthal band was removed, while decreasing the exposure of lacrimal mucosa.

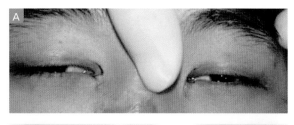

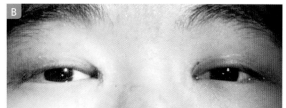

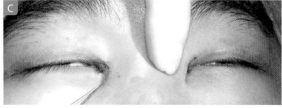

FIGURE 4-21 • Operative design in the management of depressed scar. The V-shaped incision is designed along the depressed scar.

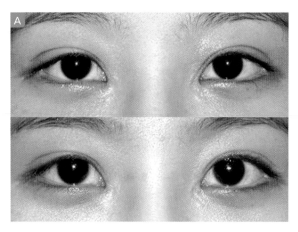

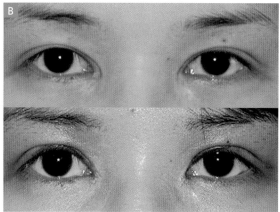

FIGURE 4-22 • In these patients, previous epicanthoplasty operations has resulted in prominent scar depressions. Both underwent reconstruction to hide the depressed scar behind the fold. The epicanthal out-folds are changed to infold.

📑 REFERENCES

1. Oh YH, Seul CH, Yoo WM : Medial epicanthoplasty using the skin redraping method. Plast Reconstr Surg 119;2:703, 2007.
2. Hwang K, Kim DJ, Hwang SH : Anatomy of lower lacrimal canaliculus relative to epicanthoplasty. J Craniofac Surg 16:949, 2005.

BLEPHAROPTOSIS

- Classification of blepharoptosis
- Preoperative assessment
- Histology of levator muscles in blepharoptosis
- Operative classification of blepharoptosis
- Operative techniques
- Other types of blepharoptosis
- Recurrence of ptosis
- Unilateral ptosis and asymmetric ptosis
- Partially ptotic eyelids
- The difficulty in accurate correction of ptosis
- Ptosis correction with general anesthesia
- Postoperative outcome and management
- Ptosis correction and double fold operation
- Upper eyelid retraction

The upper eyelid margin covers 1 to 2 mm of upper corneal limbus during primary gaze. Blepharoptosis is defined by greater than 2 mm of limbus coverage or by marginal reflex distance-1 (MRD1) less than 4 mm. Such descent of the upper eyelid can be caused by congenital or acquired deficiency in the functioning of levator palpebrae superioris or Müller's muscle.

Traditionally, corrective operations have been performed for those patients meeting the strict definition of blepharoptosis. However, these operations have found aesthetic indication even in patients who wish to have a more exposed view of the eyes. Younger patients prefer upper limbus coverage of approximately 1 mm, whereas coverage of 2 mm is more appropriate for elderly patients.

CLASSIFICATION OF BLEPHAROPTOSIS

Among many types of classifications, the classification by Beard is introduced here.

1. Congenital ptosis
a. Normal superior rectus muscle function – simple ptosis
b. Abnormal levator muscle function
c. Blepharophimosis syndrome
d. Synkinetic ptosis, Marcus-Gunn jaw winking ptosis, Misdirected third cranial nerve ptosis

2. Acquired ptosis
a. Neurogenic
b. Myogenic
c. Traumatic
d. Mechanical

3. Pseudoptosis
a. Anophthalmia, microphthalmia, phthisis bulbi
b. Hypotropia
c. Dermatochalasis

PREOPERATIVE ASSESSMENT

- Physical exam for upper corneal limbus coverage and MRD1
- Levator palpebrae superioris function
- Oculomotor function and Bell's phenomenon
- Schirmer's test and corneal sensitivity
- Synkinetic movement
- Myasthenia gravis test
- Visual acuity test
- Hering's law test
- Examination of Eyelid function

Height of palpebral fissure (FIGURE 5-1)

The palpebral fissure height is measured between the upper and lower eyelid margins at mid-pupillary line. The average fissure height is 10 mm among the Caucasian population (Fox, 1966) and 8-to-8.5 mm in the Korean population (Park et al.). A common error in evaluating the fissure height arises in patients with dermatochalasis. To evaluate the fissure height, the lax skin of the upper eyelid needs to be elevated by lifting the eyebrow. However, excessive traction on the eyebrow can inadvertently raise the upper eyelid margin as well, which should be avoided.

The palpebral fissure height is a relative measurement that can change with the position of lower eyelid margin.

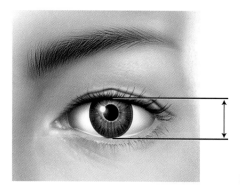

FIGURE 5-1 • Palpebral fissure height.

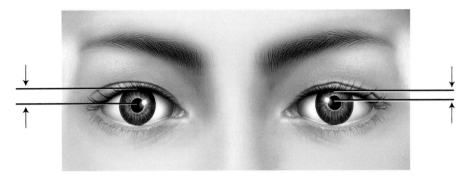

FIGURE 5-2 • The normal range for marginal reflex distance-1 (MRD1) is 3-to-5 mm. The right eye is representative of normal MRD1, whereas the MRD1 of the left eye is suggestive of blepharoptosis.

Marginal reflex distance-1 (FIGURE 5-2)

The marginal reflex distance-1 (MRD1) is defined as the distance between the corneal light reflex and the midpoint of upper eyelid margin. If the eyelid margin rests below the corneal light reflex, the distance is presented as a negative value. In Caucasian populations, the mean MRD1 was reported to be 4.5 mm. (Putterman, 1980) In the Korean population, the normal range is from 3 to 5 mm, with less than 3 mm of MRD1 indicating blepharoptosis. A 3-mm MRD1 can be associated with ptotic appearance in individuals with larger corneal diameter.

Evaluation of levator palpebrae function

The two most commonly used evaluations for levator function are the Berke method and margin limbal distance (MLB).

Berke method (FIGURE 5-3)

To eliminate any influence from the frontalis muscle, the examiner must immobilize the eyebrow onto the brow ridge with manual pressure. The patient is instructed to shift the gaze to the lowermost and uppermost positions, which will cause the eyelid margin to move in respective directions. The upper and lower positions of the eyelid margin are marked on a stationary ruler, and the distance between these to positions represent the range of motion, or excursion, of the upper eyelid. The method is easy to use in patients with upper eyelid crease. In patients without double fold, however, lax skin can hide the upper eyelid margin and require an additional hand to undrape the eyelid margin with a stylus. Thus, accurate measurement

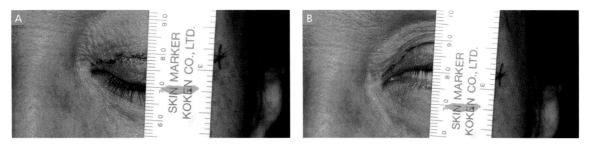

FIGURE 5-3 • Evaluation of levator function.

With the eyebrow fixed manually, the upper eyelid margin is compared between lower gaze (**A**) and upper gaze (**B**). In this patient, the left upper eyelid demonstrates 10 mm of excursion.

in the latter group of patients requires immobilization of the eyebrow as well as undraping of lax eyelid skin. When examining a crease-less eyelid, the author prefers to mentally compensate for how much of the palpebral fissure height is masked by the lax skin.

At times, examiners measure the upper eyelid excursion as the difference between the eyelid margins at closed position and at the uppermost gaze. Fact of the matter is that the upper eyelid margin assumes a much lower position with down-gaze, when compared to the position for closed eyelids. In the South Korean population, normal range for levator function is 14 to 16 mm (Park et al. 1990), whereas the normal range is 15-18 mm for Caucasian patients (Putterman, 1980). Levator function of less than 12 mm is suggestive of blepharoptosis.

Marginal limb distance (MLD) method

The marginal limb distance must also be measured with the eyebrow immobilized. The patient is instructed to bring the gaze to the uppermost extreme, and the distance is measured between the upper eyelid margin and the corneal lower limbus at 6 o'clock position. This method is useful for evaluating symmetry of levator function during blepharoptosis operation. In Caucasian population, the mean MLD is reported to be 9 mm (Putterman, 1980).

Contraindications for blepharoptosis correction

- Oculomotor nerve palsy: levator palpebrae superioris paralysis, negative Bell's phenomenon
- History of keratorefractive operation (i.e. LASIK)

- Xerophthalmia
- Decreased corneal sensitivity
- Lagophthalmos

In conditions listed above, postoperative exposure keratitis is a serious risk. As such, blepharoptosis surgery should be avoided. If it is absolutely necessary, the degree of elevation should be limited to protect the cornea.

Exposure keratitis can be a serious complication of blepharoptosis correction and can be a significant factor that deters complete correction of ptosis. There are two clinical observations related to blepharoptosis correction and exposure keratitis. The first observation is that the same extent of correction in two patients with similar degree of ptosis can result in varying degrees of lagophthalmos – due to patient factors as well as operative techniques. The second observation is that a wide variation exists in how patients tolerate what appears to the similar degree of lagophthalmos. The author has experienced extremes of these observations. In one case, a patient with complete lack of levator function had undergone correction of ptosis. Despite the levator dysfunction, the patient was able to close her eyelids in the immediate postoperative setting while achieving adequate correction of ptosis. In another patient with relatively mild ptosis, the corrective operation had resulted in the slightest lagophthalmos, which eventually led to decreased visual acuity secondary to exposure keratitis. Generally, younger patients tend do acclimate and overcome lagophthalmos and exposure keratitis better than elderly patients.

The ability to close eyelid is very important in preoperative evaluation of blepharoptosis. A proportion of ptosis patients have congenital weakness of orbicularis oculi muscle, and these patients demonstrate lagophthalmos when under anesthesia despite the presence of blepharoptosis in the awake state. Slight lagophthalmos can be present in patients with multiple blepharoplasty operations. In such cases, patients must be counseled on the possibility of postoperative lagophthalmos.

The pretarsal portion of oculi muscle is the primary motor for closing of the eyelid aperture, and it is important to preserve as much of this muscle when operating on the upper eyelid to decrease the risk of lagophthalmos.

Blepharoptosis and visual function

Congenital blepharoptosis is associated with decreased visual acuity and can be accompanied by amblyopia, strabismus, astigmatism, and myopia.

Amblyopia

The incidence of amblyopia is 3.2% in the general population, which compares to a relatively higher incidence for blepharoptosis patients (Anderson 20%, Merriam 29%, Bennish 32%). The correlation between ptosis and amblyopia becomes stronger with severity of the ptotic condition. The common types are anisometropia (13 to 15%), followed by strabismus, astigmatism, and stimulus deprivation (occlusive). Among various types, amblyopia with neither strabismus nor anisometropia is considered to be isolated ptosis. In such cases, amblyopia was present in 16.7% of patients.

Strabismus

Strabismus is a common cause of amblyopia (Lin 16%, Anderson 34%, Berke 26%). Exotropia is the most frequent type of strabismus with paralysis of superior rectus muscle present in 16%.

Astigmatism

Astigmatism is present in 45% of patients with blepharoptosis, which is about two times the incidence found in the general population. Blepharoptosis increases the contact area between the orbit and the upper eyelid, which increases uneven pressure distribution across the cornea. With-the-rule astigmatism is predominant. Correction of ptosis can change the contact area between the cornea and eyelid, with subsequent changes to astigmatism.

Myopia

The incidence is similar between blepharoptosis and general populations.

Timing of corrective operation for congenital blepharoptosis and changes in visual acuity

The optimal timing for correction of congenital blepharoptosis varies widely across the literature. A prerequisite condition for evaluating blepharoptosis is that the patient be able to communicate and cooperate with the proper examination.

Because of this, the consensus is that ptosis correction is possible after 2-3 year or 4-5 years of age.

The recommended timing of corrective operation was 3 years of age by Duke-Elder and 3-to-4 years of age by Scheie. Stallard recommended correction at 5 years of age if the child is able to see without head tilt and at 2 years of age for children who demonstrate head tilt. Fox argued that corrections were possible at any time after the age of 2. Because the fascial structure is not fully developed in children, he recommended temporary solutions using implant materials (i.e. nylon or silicone string) as slings until a definitive operation can be performed at a later time.

Whether early correction of congenital ptosis improves visual acuity has been debated by two different schools of thought. Merriam et al. reported that, at the mean age of 1.6 years, blepharoptosis correction was associated with astigmatic amblyopia in 15% of patients. To avoid this, the authors suggested operative timing after 5 years of age. However, Hornblass et al. and Lin et al. have separately reported early correction of severe congenital ptosis is effective against amblyopia. In fact, these authors have argued that delaying of operation can lead to worsening of amblyopia. Specifically, Lin et al. reported that correction of blepharoptosis between 2 months and 8 years of age was associated with decrease in the amblyopia incidence from 37.5% to 5%.

In clinical practice, it is not infrequent to observe blepharoptosis patients who, despite a severe lack of levator function, maintain visual acuity within normal range. Such patients must have had secured adequate field of vision by the utilization of the frontalis muscle through the developmental stage. In this context, congenital ptosis should be evaluated on how much it functionally interferes with securing visual field and also on how much a child is able to compensate with frontalis and without head-tilt. Delaying the operation can be a prudent approach for children who compensate appropriately and do not demonstrate any signs of amblyopia. Children with bilateral ptosis tend to acclimate to better than those with unilateral ptosis.

Both blepharoplasty and ptosis correction can lead to visual acuity changes secondary to postoperative astigmatism. This change is a consequence of decreased contact pressure on the cornea by the upper eyelid and occurs more frequently after ptosis correction than after simple blepharoplasty. In most cases, mild astigmatism can develop in most patients during the 2-3 months after the operation, with less than 10% of patients experiencing persistent astigmatism with greater than 0.3 of diopter difference after one year.

Additionally, decreased visual acuity from postoperative exposure keratitis is a serious cause for concern. The general assumption is that exposure keratitis is worse with greater amount of ptosis correction, but this is not always the case. The degree of ptosis correction does not directly correlate with increased amount of exposed cornea, and the ability to tolerate increased exposure varies widely across individual patients. All of these variable factors should be considered in the management of ptosis patients.

In order to decrease the risk of exposure keratitis, patients should apply lacrimal ointment and eye drops at nighttime. Eye patches should be considered for severe postoperative lagophthalmos.

HISTOLOGY OF LEVATOR MUSCLES IN BLEPHAROPTOSIS

Müller's muscle

- **Congenital**: Fatty infiltration is the most noticeable. Most studies have reported no significant histologic abnormality or atrophy of the myocytes. Berke et al. and Jung et al. have reported lack of atrophy in 2/3 of patients and mild atrophy in 1/3 of patients.
- **Acquired**: The muscle fibers are relatively abundant (Berke). However, the muscle fibers are atrophied and demonstrates degenerative changes.

Levator palpebrae superioris muscle

The most common cause of congenital blepharoptosis is dystrophy of the levator muscle, which is demonstrated by atrophy and fibrosis on histologic examination (Hueck. 70-95% atrophy and 42% fibrosis). The pattern of atrophy includes hyaline degeneration and vacuolization of muscle fibers. In severe cases of blepharoptosis, it is not uncommon to observe complete absence of muscle cells. Fatty infiltration has been reported to be found in 25% of cases. Senile ptosis is caused by aponeurotic disinsertion but is also accompanied by muscular degeneration in a large number of cases. The degree of abnormality in the striated muscle correlates well with the dysfunction in levator function.

In acquired ptosis, striated fibers of levator muscle appear normal. (Berke et al.)

Levator aponeurosis

The mean thickness of aponeurosis is 0.2 mm in patients with ptosis, which is not a distinguishing feature compared to normal population.

OPERATIVE CLASSIFICATION OF BLEPHAROPTOSIS

The author categorizes various types of blepharoptosis by operative techniques required: biologic versus mechanical. These two categories differ significantly in the amount of advancement that is required, and as such, it is important to understand the differences in the mechanism.

Biologic ptosis
- Congenital ptosis
- Traumatic ptosis

Biologic ptosis encompasses all manner of dystrophy of the levator complex, as represented by biologic and histologic abnormalities (fibrosis, hypotrophy, dystrophy, fatty infiltration, etc.). Such structural changes of levator complex can be found in congenital ptosis as well as traumatic ptosis (post-trauma fibrotic change).

In contrast to senile ptosis, congenital ptosis demonstrates distinct histologic abnormalities of the levator muscle and therefore can be classified as a biologic ptosis. Myopathic problems can also be found in post-blepharoplasty ptosis, which is caused by fibrosis or scarring of the levator complex (aponeurosis, Müller's muscle, or levator muscle). In a predominant majority of cases, traumatic ptosis is similar to congenital ptosis in histologic findings, operative solutions, and postoperative complication. However, traumatic ptosis can cause disinsertion of aponeurosis without any scarring, which would be considered mechanical ptosis.

Mechanical ptosis

Mechanical ptosis refers to disinsertion or dehiscence of the aponeurosis without any structural or functional changes to the motor component of the levator complex.

It encompasses aponeurotic ptosis and traumatic aponeurotic disinsertion.

No single case of ptosis is 100% mechanical in nature. In senile ptosis, degenerative changes can be observed as primary cause in as many cases as aponeurotic disinsertion. Even if the main cause of ptosis is aponeurotic failure, Müller's muscle can undergo atrophy, attenuation, fibrosis, and/or fatty infiltration.

The changes to the musculature in mechanical ptosis are relatively mild when compared to that of biologic ptosis. Because of this, mechanical ptosis requires relatively lower amount of tissue advancement than required for biologic ptosis.

Aponeurotic ptosis

Involutional ptosis belongs to aponeurotic ptosis.

Aponeurotic ptosis is caused by the stretching, thinning, dehiscence, or disinsertion of the aponeurosis, which prevents the transmission of muscular force to the tarsal plate and the rest of the upper eyelid and eventually leads to atrophy of Müller's or levator muscle.

In aponeurotic ptosis, the defect is between the terminal portion of aponeurosis and the tarsal plate. Because of this, the levator maintains relatively good function, even in severe examples of mechanical ptosis (FIGURE 5-5).

In determining the amount of advancement required at the time of operation, the two main variables to consider are the degree of ptosis and the levator function. The levator function correlates with the range of motion, which implies changes to elasticity, fibrosis, atrophy, fatty infiltration of the muscle itself. Therefore, a patient with minimal levator function would require more advancement than would be suspected purely on the basis of ptosis severity. In contrast, a patient with a full range of motion will probably require a lot less advancement even if the ptosis is severe.

The biologic changes observed in aponeurotic ptosis are incidental, and the main etiology is mechanical changes (disinsertion or dehiscence). Even severe degree of mechanical ptosis portends good prognosis because the underlying levator musculature is intact and able to lift the tarsal plate and upper eyelid, once the physical linkage between the aponeurosis and tarsal plate is restored. In most cases, the amount of advancement required for aponeurotic ptosis is far less that required for biologic ptosis. However, not every case of ptosis in an elderly patient can be assumed to be mechanical in nature. It is still possible to observe biologic ptosis in the older population. Senile ptosis can arise as a combination of biologic and mechanical causes in patients with congenitally weak levator function. Because of these complicated factors, calculation of advancement should take into account both the degree of ptosis and the levator function.

Etiology

- Involutional ptosis
- Post-blepharoplasty complication
- Blepharochalasis
- Blepharospasm
- Long-term contact lens use
- Dermatitis leading to habitual rubbing of the eyelids
- Ophthalmic operation (for cataract or glaucoma)
- Pregnancy
- Severe edema
- Hyperthyroidism
- Traumatic disruption of the aponeurosis

The most common type of aponeurotic ptosis is involutional ptosis in the elderly, followed by long-term contact lens use. It can also be observed in patients with

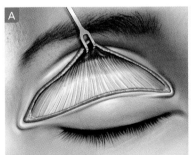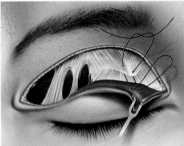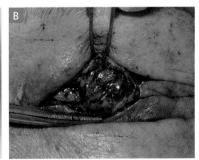

FIGURE 5-4 ● **A.** Dehiscence of aponeurosis is repaired and advanced in a single step. **B.** Intraoperative photograph of a defect between the aponeurosis and the Müller's muscle.

dermatologic disorders who frequently rub the eyelids to relieve pruritus, which can lead to degeneration or stretching of the aponeurosis. Traumatic or iatrogenic injury to the aponeurosis is also a cause **(FIGURE 5-4)**.

In addition to those above, severe swelling of the eyelid can also lead to apo-neurotic ptosis, which can caused after facial soft tissue injury in motor vehicle collision, chemotherapy, pregnancy (preeclampsia), and hyperthyroidism. It is impor-tant to note that iatrogenic injury to the aponeurosis at the time of blepharoplasty does not lead to immediate postoperative ptosis because Müller's muscle remains intact. Over time, however, Müller's muscle can attenuate, and ptosis can develop many years after the initial blepharoplasty. Because of this, the aponeurosis is sig-nificantly thin in aponeurotic ptosis but is relatively intact in congenital ptosis. Ophthalmic operations for cataract and glaucoma are associated with aponeurosis dehiscence in 3-13% of cases. This complication may be caused by the intraopera-tive use of bridle suture and/or postoperative inflammation.

In most cases, history can differentiate between aponeurotic and congenital ptosis. Exceptions arise in those patients with subclinical variants of congenital ptosis, which was compensated by frontalis muscle use at an earlier age and which was no longer compensated in later years. It is also possible that senile ptosis devel-ops in a patient who has a congenital ptosis.

Clinical characteristics of senile ptosis include asymmetric development of ptosis across the eyes, progressively worsening ptosis, and lack of accompanying oculo-motor dysfunction or amblyopia. Occasionally, senile ptosis requires work up for myasthenia gravis and Horner's syndrome.

Examination characteristics

In contrast to congenital ptosis, aponeurotic ptosis is associated with preserved levator function relative to the degree of ptosis itself **(FIGURE 5-5)**. In congenital ptosis, the fibrotic levator muscle is less elastic. Because of this, the upper eyelid margin can actually appear elevated with lower gaze (lid lag) **(FIGURE 5-6)**. In apo-neurotic ptosis, lower gaze is associated with significant ptosis of the upper eyelid margin. As such, patients with aponeurotic ptosis complain of fatigue and even headache during downgaze and experience significant difficulty walking down stairs **(FIGURE 5-7)**. The presence of sunken eyelid is most likely due to retracted aponeuro-sis drawing the orbital fat upward or due to the effects of compensating eyebrow. It

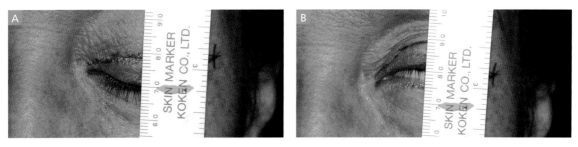

FIGURE 5-5 • Levator function of senile ptosis patient.
this is the same patient from **FIGURE 5-3**. **A.** At lowermost gaze, the upper eyelid margin is at 70 mm. **B.** At uppermost gaze, the margin is at 80 mm. The levator function is 10 mm, which is more than adequate considering severity of the ptosis itself.

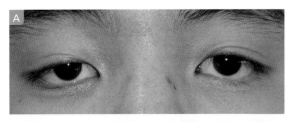
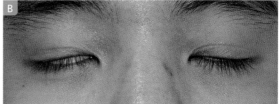
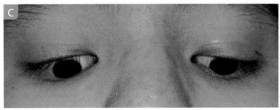

FIGURE 5-6 • Lid lag in a patient with congenital ptosis of the right eye. The right eyelid margin appears higher than the left eyelid margin with down gaze.

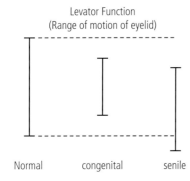

Levator Function
(Range of motion of eyelid)

Normal   congenital   senile

FIGURE 5-7 • Comparison of levator function.
The bar ends represent the position of upper eyelid margin from upward to downward gaze. In congenital ptosis, the ptotic eyelid does not lower as much as a normal eyelid (lid lag). In aponeurotic ptosis, the upper eyelid margin can be much lower than that of the normal eyelid.

is possible to observe high fold or loss of fold, as well as faintness of the crease just above the upper border of tarsal plate (FIGURE 5-8). Another characteristic of senile ptosis is the lateral shifting of the tarsal plate due to the disinsertion of the medial portion of aponeurosis.

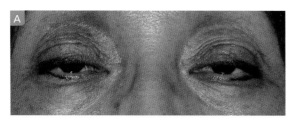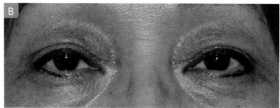

FIGURE 5-8 • Senile or involutional ptosis.
A. Preoperatively, the ptotic eyelids demonstrate hollowness. The eyelid crease is faint but located high. **B.** The ptosis correction restores fullness to the eyelid and lowers the eyelid crease. Levator advancement amount is 6 mm.

TABLE 5-1 • Comparison between congenital and aponeurotic ptosis (**FIGURE 5-8, 5-9**)

	Congenital	Aponeurotic
Levator dysfunction	Severe	Mild
Lower gaze	Lid lag may be present or absent	Ptotic eyelid margin
Visual dysfunction (amblyopia, astigmatism, or strabismus)	Higher than average incidence	Average incidence
Complex ptosis (Oculomotor dysfunction, synkinesis)	Possible	None
Double fold	Absent in most cases	High fold or loss of fold
Clinical course	Stable	Progressive
Miscellaneous detail		Sunken, thin eyelid Lateral shifting of tarsal plate

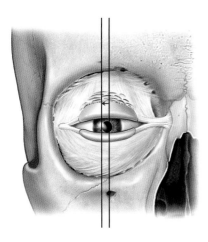

FIGURE 5-9 • Disinsertion of the medial aponeurosis leads to lateral shifting of the tarsal plate in senile ptosis.

Operative techniques for aponeurotic ptosis

- Levator advancement
- Müller plication and levator advancement
- Levator complex plication

Congenital ptosis

Congenital ptosis is caused by the hypoplasia of the levator complex. Histology of the Müller's and levator muscles demonstrates atrophy, dystrophy, fibrosis, rarefaction, and fatty infiltration. In severe congenital ptosis, the muscle fiber of levator muscle has an irregular appearance or is absent. Congenital ptosis is autosomal dominant in 10% of cases. According to Reeh et al., superior rectus muscle paresis is present in 16% of cases.

Traumatic or post-blepharoplasty ptosis can be associated with fibrosis of the levator muscle, which needs to be distinguished from injury limited to aponeurosis. The management of such fibrotic changes must take into account the decrease in levator function, as is the case for congenital ptosis. Such traumatic ptosis is similar to congenital ptosis in both the operative techniques required and potential postoperative complications such as lid lag.

Indicated operative techniques

- Müller advancement
- Levator complex plication
- Levator shortening surgery
- CFS advancement and levator shortening combination surgery
- Frontalis transfer

Aponeurosis surgery has been suggested for the management of mild congenital ptosis. However, aponeurosis surgery is associated with high rates of recurrent ptosis. The author does not recommend aponeurosis surgery for congenital cases.

Blepharoptosis correction techniques can be classified as follows:

Blepharoptosis operative techniques

Levator complex surgery (FIGURE 5-10)

- Aponeurosis surgery
- Müller tuck and aponeurosis surgery
- Under-through levator complex plication surgery
- Levator shortening surgery

Check ligament (or Conjoint fascial sheath) and levator shortening combination surgery

Frontalis surgery

- Frontalis transfer
- Frontalis sling

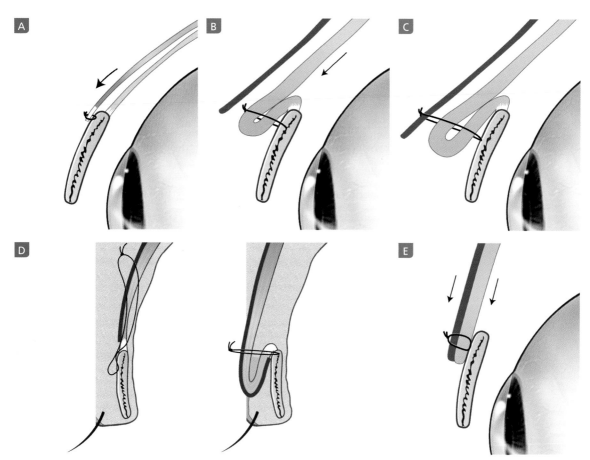

FIGURE 5-10 • Illustration of various ptosis correction techniques with levator complex.
A. Levator advancement. **B.** Müller tuck. **C.** Müller tuck and aponeurosis advancement. **D.** Under through technique of levator plication technique.
E. Levator shortening surgery.

OPERATIVE TECHNIQUES

Levator aponeurosis advancement

Aponeurosis advancement is an effective way of addressing aponeurotic ptosis. Aponeurotic ptosis is different from congenital ptosis in many aspects, and as such, the treatment must differ for each type of ptosis.

The main pathology behind aponeurotic ptosis is the stretching, dehiscence, or disinsertion of the aponeurosis with the ensuing attenuation of the Müller's muscle. Thus, congenital ptosis represents an abnormal biological muscle quality, and aponeurotic ptosis represents mechanical abnormality.

The ideal operative correction must reflect proper understanding of the mechanism behind aponeurotic ptosis. The aponeurosis should be advanced to compensate for both the deficit created by dehiscence and the attenuation of Müller's muscle.

Compared to correction of congenital ptosis, aponeurotic ptosis requires relatively conservative approach and mild advancement. Whereas congenital ptosis requires large tissue advancements (3-4 times the length of ptosis to be corrected), aponeurotic ptosis is corrected by conservative procedures with far less advancement, that is to say stretched or dehisced aponeurosis of involutional ptosis does not require large advancements. In contrast, large advancements are required for muscular atrophy in the absence of aponeurotic defect.

Regional anesthetic is preferred over general anesthesia because the patient is able to cooperate with instructions to open and close the eyelids, which is essential to evaluating the ptosis and symmetry of the palpebral fissure in unilateral cases. It is important to be wary of local anesthetic agents temporarily blocking the Müller's and levator muscles. It is also possible that an anesthetic agent can selective block the orbicularis muscle, which can cause the palpebral fissure to assume a wider aperture. Epinephrine can activate Müller's muscle and cause the lid to be retracted. Because of these reason, it is important to minimize potential changes in the lid position from anesthetics.

Operative details

After preoperative consultation and designing of the eyelid incision, the regional anesthetic is administered with the patient under light sedation. The author uses 1% lidocaine mixed with 1:100,000 epinephrine to block supraorbital nerve,

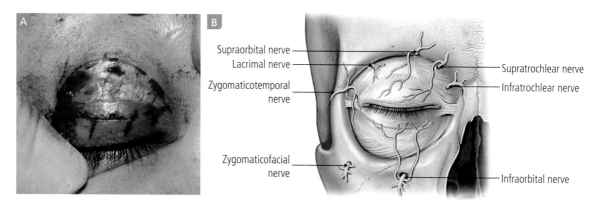

Supraorbital nerve
Lacrimal nerve
Zygomaticotemporal nerve
Zygomaticofacial nerve
Supratrochlear nerve
Infratrochlear nerve
Infraorbital nerve

FIGURE 5-11 • **A.** Sensory nerve branches travel inferiorly over the orbital septum. **B.** Periorbital nerve branches.

supratrochlear nerve, infratrochlear nerve, and lacrimal nerve. The supraorbital and supratrochlear nerves are blocked by the injection of 1.0-1.5 ml of anesthetic at and medial to the supraorbital foramen. The lacrimal nerve is blocked 1 cm superior to the lateral canthal tendon. An alternative to blocking the lacrimal nerve is to inject relatively copious amount of local anesthetic in the lateral portion of the eyelid skin, which is safe to do because anesthetic far to the lateral portion does not change the eyelid position. Anesthetic agents should be injected deep to the orbicularis muscle, i.e. in the retro-orbicularis oculi fat or around the orbital septum, as the sensory nerve branches travel just superficial to the septum **(FIGURE 5-11)**.

In addition to the regional blocks, the skin incision along the eyelid crease is injected with a local anesthetic using 30G needle. Superior to the crease, the skin is anesthetized without any epinephrine. Inferior to the crease, the anesthetic solution may contain epinephrine because there is no Müller's muscle at this level.

Intraoperatively, additional anesthetic is injected in the plane just superficial to the tarsal plates. It is important that this portion of anesthetic does not reach the pretarsal orbicularis oculi muscle. If necessary, another injection is administered around the orbital septum, which is separated from the Müller's muscle by the orbital fat.

Upon anesthesia, the skin is incised along the eyelid crease and carried past the orbicularis muscle. The orbital septum is identified and separated away from the levator aponeurosis. If the patient expresses discomfort at this point, lidocaine without epinephrine is injected in the central portion of the septum and tarsal plate to be advanced, as the sensory nerve travels inferiorly along the orbital septum. Tetracaine eye drop is also helpful when applied to exposed tissue surfaces and orbital septum. It is possible that, despite careful use, anesthetic agent results in asymmetric eyelid height. If the asymmetry is great, the lidocaine without epinephrine can be injected to bring down the eyelid with higher position. If the difference is mild, the operator can take this into consideration while correcting for the advancement.

Other factors which influence the shape and position of upper eyelid include hematoma formation, traumatic handling of tissue, and edema. Prolonged operative time can lead to edema, which can decrease the ability to raise the eyelids. Because of this, it is advantageous to complete the operation in shorter duration.

Upon exposure, the aponeurosis is advanced to account for the degree of aponeurosis stretching or dehiscence, the degree of Müller's muscle stretching, and the degree of overall ptosis. The advanced portion of aponeurosis is attached 2 mm below the superior border of the tarsal plate using 6-0 nylon. Three mattress sutures are required.

 WAIT A MINUTE!

WHY FIX THE APONEUROSIS AT 2 MM BELOW THE SUPERIOR BORDER OF TARSAL PLATE?

The peripheral arterial arcade runs along the superior 1-mm border of the tarsal plate. As such, placement of the suture along the topmost edge can result in loss of hemostasis. However, placement of sutures well below the 2-mm position can result in ectropion.

The connective tissue and fat located anterior to the tarsal plate is excised to allow adhesion between the plate and the advanced aponeurosis. The pretarsal fat is especially abundant medially. The suture should be placed through a partial thickness of the tarsal plate, as to prevent the advanced aponeurosis from being pulled upwards, which would represent recurrence of ptosis. In fact, the author believes the failure to secure the aponeurosis onto the tarsal plate is the most common cause of recurrent ptosis.

Evaluation of the lid position should be performed in both the recumbent and sitting positions. When evaluating the eyelid position, the operator must pay attention to the symmetry of the eyebrows as well – asymmetry may signal compensation for one of the eyelids.

Ptosis should be corrected such that, ultimately, the eyelid margin is covering the top 1-to-1.5 mm of the upper limbus. However, it is important to understand that the eyelid margin usually lowers by a little over the course of a few months. Hence, slight overcorrection of ptosis is a prudent measure. Severe ptosis is associated with significantly elevated tension, and this requires more overcorrection than the usual 1 mm. In the elderly or in patients with xerophthalmia, undercorrection is recommended both in terms of aesthetics and function.

The probability of ptosis recurrence is dependent on the choice of technique and the number of fixation sutures used. Generally, recurrence is considered to be more common for aponeurosis advancement than for Müller tuck or levator shortening.

The aponeurosis begins at Whitnall's ligament and has a vertical length of 12 mm. Its mean thickness of 0.2 mm, and it is thinner proximally. As such, it is inadvisable to dissect and advance more than 10 mm of the aponeurosis. Additionally, aponeurotic ptosis is a result of the ongoing aging process. As such, slight overcorrection is helpful in "future proofing" against further changes.

The method of anesthesia greatly influences the success of ptosis correction

In contrast to general anesthesia, local anesthetics are helpful in assessing eyelid height during the operation, especially for unilateral ptosis. If local anesthesia injection does not change the lid position, the operator can place a higher level of confidence in the intraoperative examination and, therefore, the intraoperative progress. Here, the author reviews the anesthetic method.

Effects of local anesthetic
Local anesthetics such as lidocaine and bupivacaine have the following effects:
1. Paralyses Müller's and levator muscles and decreases upper eyelid function.
2. Paralyses orbicularis muscle, which slightly elevates the upper eyelid.
3. The volume of injection causes edema, which decreases the ability to elevate the eyelid.
4. Epinephrine activates Müller's muscle and increases the eyelid height. The amount of elevation has been reported to be 1.0 mm after 10 minutes of

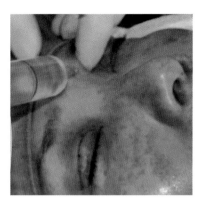

FIGURE 5-12 • Regional block.
The left index finger is used to palpate the orbital rim, and the anesthetic is infiltrated to the orbital rim to minimize the effects of anesthetic on the levator muscle.

epinephrine instillation (Bartley, 1995) and 1-to-1.5 mm (Brown).

These effects of local anesthetic are accentuated by the sensitiveness of muscle. In patients with mild ptosis (i.e. preserved levator function), the bare minimal of local anesthesia should be used. The inverse is also true; liberal use of anesthesia does not interfere with eyelid height in severe ptosis.

Regional block

A mixture of 1% lidocaine and 1:100,000 epinephrine is used to block the supraorbital nerve, supratrochlear nerve, infratrochlear nerve, and the lacrimal nerve. The lacrimal nerve is blocked 0.5 to 1.0 ml superior to the lateral canthal tendon. An alternative to blocking the lacrimal nerve is to inject relatively copious amount of local anesthetic in the lateral portion of the eyelid skin. This is considered relatively safe because the anesthetic does not change the eyelid position in this area. The sensory nerve branches travel in the plane superficial to the septum. Because of this anesthetic agents should be injected deep to the orbicularis muscle. The operator's free hand is used to palpate the orbital rim, and the anesthetic is infiltrated to the rim to block the supraorbital nerve and supratrochlear nerve. Such method limits the anesthetic effect on levator complex (FIGURE 5-12).

Local anesthesia

The tissue deep to incision line (i.e. upper tarsal border) is the most sensitive to local anesthesia, and local anesthesia should be avoided in this area. This is especially important in the case of secondary operations where the orbicularis muscle has

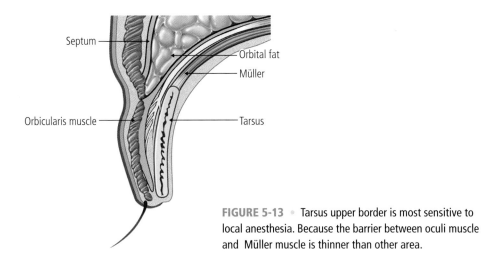

FIGURE 5-13 • Tarsus upper border is most sensitive to local anesthesia. Because the barrier between oculi muscle and Müller muscle is thinner than other area.

already been excised **(FIGURE 5-13)**.

Superior to the crease, the skin is anesthetized without any epinephrine. Inferior to the crease, a limited amount of lidocaine and epinephrine mixture is injected. Intraoperatively, a small amount of lidocaine without epinephrine can be injected in the pretarsal tissue. Anesthetic eye drops can be applied to the conjunctiva to reduce the discomfort.

Indication for levator aponeurosis advancement

Aponeurosis advancement is most commonly used to correct aponeurotic ptosis. It is effective in patients who maintain levator function greater than 8 mm, and has been reported to be effective even in congenital ptosis. However, the aponeurosis is not a robust structure, and some surgeons avoid using aponeurosis advancement even for aponeurotic ptosis – especially in the case of degenerative aponeurosis. The author does not use aponeurosis advancement in even the mildest form of congenital ptosis.

What are levator aponeurosis plication and levator aponeurosis advancement?

Levator aponeurosis plication does not dissect the aponeurosis from the Müller's muscle, whereas the dissection of aponeurosis leads to advancement of the aponeurosis. This technical distinction is important because there is a significant

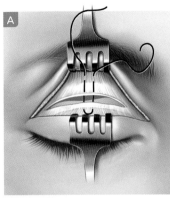
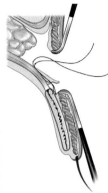

FIGURE 5-14 • Aponeurosis advancement for aponeurotic ptosis.
A. Illustration. **B.** Pre/postoperative photographs of patients with aponeurotic ptosis who underwent aponeurosis advancement.

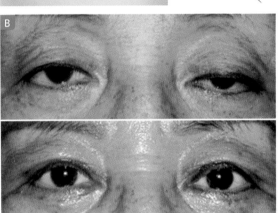
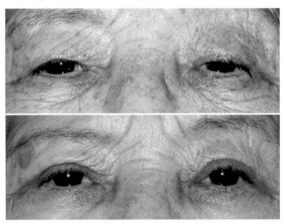

difference in the level of adhesion between the two methods. The aponeurosis is a gliding membrane with low levels of adhesion. The uninjured aponeurosis and good gliding property is less likely to adhere to the tarsal plate, and recurrence of ptosis is more likely. In contrast, trauma to the site of fixation between aponeurosis and the plate will create enough adhesion to correct the ptosis without recurrence. Hence, plication is associated with unpredictable recurrence. Historically, most studies on levator plication have reported unsatisfactory results. The author does not use aponeurosis plication. In his book, Fox also mentioned that he had abandoned the technique because of unpredictable outcomes. The author prefers the under through technique over the traditional method.

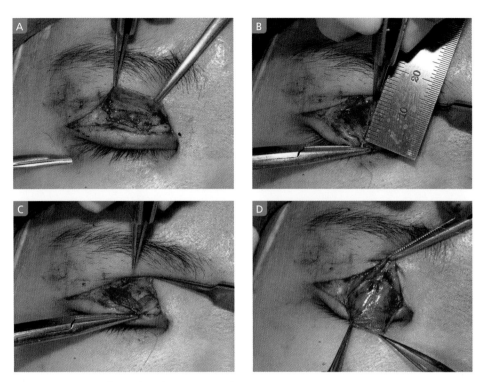

FIGURE 5-15 • Müller tuck and aponeurosis advancement.
A. The dissection plane between aponeurosis and Müller's muscle. **B.** The advancement length is measured from the tarsal plate to Müller's muscle. **C.** The Müller's muscle is sutured. **D.** The aponeurosis is advanced.

Müller muscle plication and levator aponeurosis advancement

Müller muscle plication was introduced by Saijo from Japan. The author combines aponeurosis advancement with this technique, as Müller muscle plication by itself has been inadequate in preventing recurrence of ptosis.

The combination of Müller muscle plication and levator aponeurosis advancement provides advancement of a tissue complex that is more robust than the advancement of either aponeurosis or Müller's muscle alone. The addition of aponeurosis advancement prevents stretching, atrophy, or dehiscence of the muscle. Postoperative outcomes are more predictable when these two techniques are used in combination.

Indication

• Aponeurotic ptosis – technique is effective regardless of the degree of ptosis.

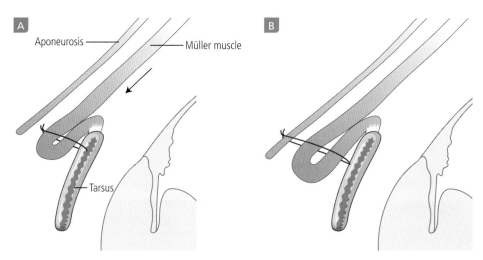

FIGURE 5-16 • **A.** Müller plication. **B.** Müller plication and aponeurosis advancement.

- Mild-to-moderate degree of congenital ptosis
- Traumatic ptosis

This combination technique is effective in aponeurotic ptosis regardless of the degree of ptosis. It is also indicated for mild-to-moderate congenital ptosis (less than 2-mm of ptosis), as well as used widely for iatrogenic or traumatic ptosis (**FIGURE 5-16**). However, greater than 3 mm of congenital ptosis is better addressed by other techniques such as levator shortening.

Operative details

The initial stage of operation is similar to that of aponeurosis advancement operation, which includes skin incision, orbicularis incision, and dissection of the aponeurosis from the Müller's muscle. It is important not to injure the peripheral arterial arcade, which is located in the top 1 mm of the tarsal plate, anterior to Müller's muscle, and which can easily be injured during the dissection. Once separated from the aponeurosis, Müller's muscle is plicated and the aponeurosis is advanced. Both are fixed onto the tarsal plate. The length of advancement can be the same or different between the two structures. The author is of the opinion that the amount of advancement should be commensurate between the aponeurosis and the muscle in order to decrease the risk of early operative failure from muscle stretching. Because the aponeurosis is not an elastic structure, however, some argue that

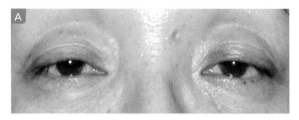
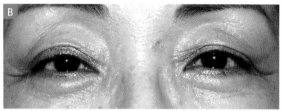

FIGURE 5-17 • Müller tuck and aponeurosis advancement in senile ptosis.

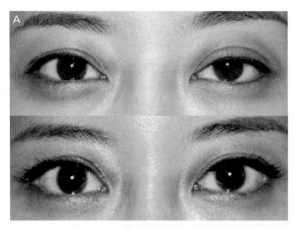
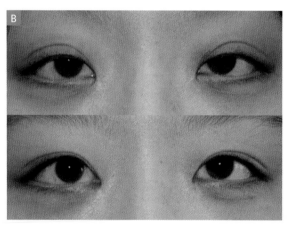

FIGURE 5-18 • Müller tuck and aponeurosis advancement in congenital ptosis.

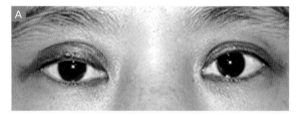
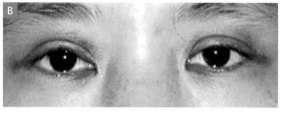

FIGURE 5-19 • Müller tuck and aponeurosis advancement in iatrogenic ptosis.

limiting the aponeurosis advancement allows for smoother eyelid movement as well as decreased risk of lid lag and lagophthalmos. Another convenient method of separating aponeurosis from Müller's muscle is the excision of the distal portion of aponeurosis.

Depending on the degree of ptosis, the Müller's muscle is plicated and fixated on the tarsal plate about 2 mm from the upper border, using 7-0 or 6-0 nylon.

At each suture point, it is possible to fixate the aponeurosis at the time of muscle

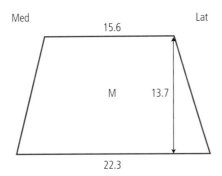

Med   15.6   Lat

M   13.7

22.3

FIGURE 5-20 • Müller muscle (whang).

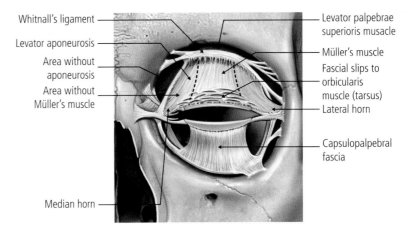

Whitnall's ligament

Levator aponeurosis

Area without aponeurosis

Area without Müller's muscle

Levator palpebrae superioris musacle

Müller's muscle

Fascial slips to orbicularis muscle (tarsus)

Lateral horn

Capsulopalpebral fascia

Median horn

FIGURE 5-21 • Müller muscle and levator aponeurosis.

plication. However, the author prefers to finish the row of sutures (3 to 5 stitches) for muscle plication first and work on the aponeurosis advancement as a separate step. This is because simultaneous fixation of the two layers makes it difficult to visualize the adjacent fixation site **(FIGURE 5-17, 5-18, 5-19)**.

The Müller's muscle is an involuntary muscle. While closing and opening of the eyelid appears to be under volition at all times, the eyelid aperture has a strong autonomous component. Total excision of Müller's muscle (e.g. levator resection) should only be considered for serious conditions. The normal range of length for Müller is 10-14 mm (Hwang 13.7 mm, Beard 10-12 mm), with a mean thickness of 0.7 ± 0.5 mm **(FIGURE 5-20)**. A full advancement of the Müller's muscle leads to a 2-mm elevation of the eyelid margin. Complete resection of Müller's muscle for retracted eyelids lowers the eyelid margin by about the same amount.

Compared to levator resection, both the aponeurosis advancement and the Müller tuck combination offer the advantage of requiring less anesthesia and thus allows for accurate assessment of the eyelid position. Also, there is less intraoperative injury and/or structural disruption of the levator muscle, Müller's muscle, and orbital septum. For example, it is possible to undo the plication in the middle of the operation if the operator suspects the local anesthetic to be interfering with the evaluation. Such maneuver is not possible in the case of levator resection.

 WAIT A MINUTE!

APONEUROSIS PLICATION VS. MÜLLER PLICATION

The term "plication" refers to the technique of mobilizing tissue by the means of folding the tissue without any dissection from underlying tissue. Keeping this in mind, why is it that Müller plication is used widely, while aponeurosis plication is not practiced?

The author believes this to be a reflection on the nature of the tissue material under comparison: Müller's muscle vs. aponeurosis. The levator aponeurosis is a type of fascia and covered with a sheath for gliding action. As such, it is difficult for the aponeurosis to adhere to itself. In contrast, Müller's muscle is a tissue that adheres well to adjacent tissue. This difference in adhesion quality is what determines the outcome of ptosis operation. As pointed by Anderson, aponeurosis plication does not consistently undergo tissue adhesion because of the lack of raw surface. If the aponeurosis is traumatized or it is thinner than usual, the chance for adhesion is higher. Aponeurosis plication remains a footnote in the history of ptosis operations.

Levator complex plication

Levator complex plication and the under-through plication technique

The traditional levator plication technique has been avoided because postoperative outcome were extremely variable. (Method 1, **FIGURE 5-22**) The author uses a modification of this technique for mild cases of ptosis, which provides a predictable postoperative outcome. (Method 2, **FIGURE 5-23**) The author refers to the method as "under-through technique of levator complex plication) because the suture passes under and through the Müller's muscle. The main distinction in this technique is that the plication does not only involve the aponeurosis but also the Müller's muscle and the levator muscle.

Two major differences between the techniques is the method by which the adhesion forms 1) in the aponeurosis and 2) in the Müller's muscle.

Levator complex plication method #1 – Plication above the aponeurosis

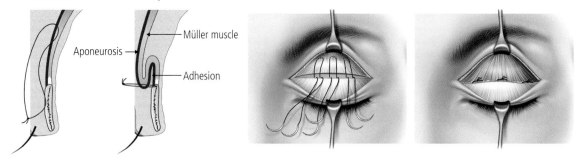

FIGURE 5-22 • The plication suture is above the aponeurosis, which does not provide a consistent rate of adhesion.

Levator complex plication method #2 – Under through technique

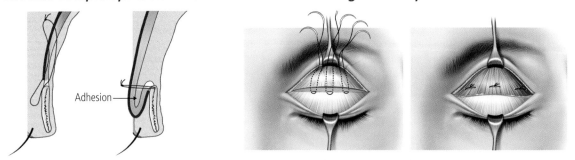

FIGURE 5-23 • The plication suture travels under and through the Müller's muscle, which forces the Müller's muscle to adhere to itself in the plication fold. This creates for a more consistent adhesion.

Under-through technique of levator complex plication (FIGURE 5-24)

The advantage of this technique is that the lack of dissection between the tissue layers (i.e. aponeurosis, Müller's muscle, and conjunctiva) decreases the need for local anesthetics, the risk of hematoma, and the operative time. In ptosis correction, any strategy that decreases operative time is welcomed because shorter operative times equates to less of edema interference with eyelid evaluation. Because the structures are mobilized en-bloc, the outcomes are more robust with the exception of the levator shortening technique.

Compared to levator shortening, the under-through technique does not require

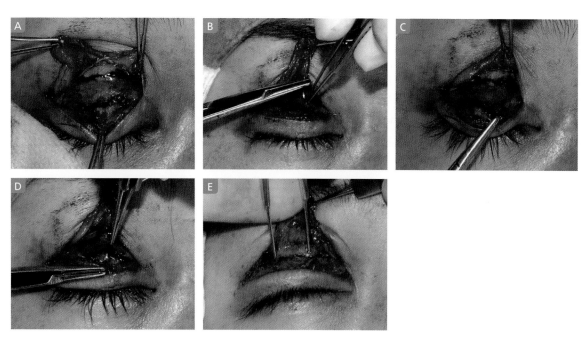

FIGURE 5-24 • Under-through levator complex plication technique.
The desired advancement is 9 mm. **A.** Top line – 7 mm above the upper border of tarsal plate. Bottom line – 2 mm below the upper border of tarsal plate. **B.** From the top line, the suture needle enters the aponeurosis passes under in the plane between the Müller's muscle and conjunctiva. **C.** At the bottom line, the needle is brought out perpendicularly while taking a partial-thickness bite of the tarsal plate. **D.** The needle is driven in the reverse direction and in the plane between aponeurosis and Müller's muscle. **E.** The plicated levator complex.

separation of the aponeurosis and Müller's muscle from the upper border of tarsal plate and conjunctiva. This allows intraoperative evaluation of the eyelid position at any time during the operation, which is not possible in certain portions of the levator shortening operation. The disadvantages of this technique is that the Müller's muscle advancement is not exactly full-thickness and that the volume effect of the plication requires few millimeters of extra advancement.

What is the mechanistic difference between the traditional plication technique and the under-through technique?

The difference is in the adhesion. The aponeurosis is a smooth gliding tissue and is resistant to postoperative fibrosis. The adhesion between aponeurosis and tarsal plate or the adhesion to aponeurosis itself is not consistent, and recurrence of ptosis is not predictable. This also is true of rarefied aponeurosis. For this reason, Fox (1979), Harris and Dorzback (1975), and Berlin and Vestal (1989) have all reported disappointment for aponeurosis plication. However, few have reported satisfactory outcomes for senile and aponeurotic ptosis (John et al. and Liu).

Aponeurosis plication has been reported to be effective for milder cases of congenital ptosis. (Burman and Ibrar Hussain) However, the author's experience has been disappointing even in mild cases of congenital ptosis.

The outcome is dependent on which structure is plicated. The under-through technique is similar to Müller plication because the Müller muscle is plicated in both techniques.

Levator shortening

The term levator shortening can be considered as levator complex shortening, which includes the aponeurosis, Müller's muscle, and the levator muscle. For severe ptosis, the levator muscle proper will be shortened, but shortening of the Müller muscle can also be considered shortening of the levator complex, which leads to a minor degree of confusion in terminology (FIGURE 5-25). Some have proposed designating shortening operations without levator muscle excision to be called "Müller and aponeurosis shortening" to clarify the distinction. However, Müller's muscle and levator muscle do not exist in a distinct anatomic zones but interdigitate with each other. Because of this anatomic ambiguity, it is difficult to know whether an operation shortened just Müller's muscle or incorporated the levator muscle at times. Regardless of the distinction, the operative details are the same in both scenarios, and both operations can be called levator shortening operation.

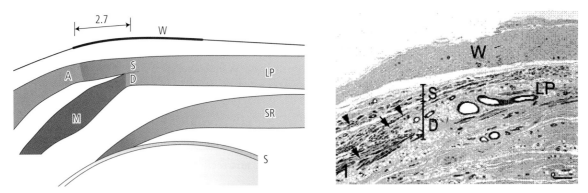

FIGURE 5-25 • The junction between Müller muscle and levator muscle contains both smooth muscle (arrow) and striated muscle (arrowhead) cells.

LP: levator aponeurosis, S: superficial, D: deep, M: Müller's muscle, SR: superior rectus. (Histology reprinted with permission from Hwang)

Operative details

Design

The skin incision is designed at the desired height, while keeping in mind that ptosis will correction will elevate the eyelid margin and lessen the distance to the eyelid crease. This change in crease height is greater in the center and less towards the medial and lateral portions of the eyelid. In order to simulate the shape of the eyelid crease after the ptosis correction, the eyebrows are fixed with an available hand. The patient is instructed to open the eyes widely and the crease is drawn with the stylus. This is not feasible in severe cases of ptosis, however.

Anesthesia

Local anesthesia is performed using a mixture of 1% lidocaine and 1/100,000 epinephrine. Because levator shortening is performed for ptosis patients with severely limited levator function, the anesthetic agent is less likely to interfere with intraoperative evaluation of eyelid position. Therefore, the author recommends liberal use of anesthetics for this operation.

Skin incision and dissection

Upon skin incision and opening the orbicularis muscle, the aponeurosis is exposed after being separated from the septum. These initial steps are the same to those discussed in previous techniques. Diluted lidocaine-normal saline solution (1/3 concentration) is used to dissect the space between Müller's muscle and conjunctiva. An alternative method is to apply tetracaine eye drops into the conjunctiva and to use pure normal saline solution for dissection. The levator complex (aponeurosis and Müller's muscle) is incised and separated away from the tarsal plate, while taking care not to disturb the peripheral arterial arcade. The complex is then dissected superiorly, away from the conjunctiva underneath. At this time, it is important not to puncture the conjunctiva. If the conjunctiva is punctured, the conjunctival defect must be repaired in a meticulous fashion, or the injury can lead to the formation of mucoid cyst. If large advancements are required, the horn might be resected bilaterally. More often than not, however, it is possible that resection of the lateral horn alone might be sufficient because the medial horn is relatively elastic. Superiorly, the dissection is carried out as much as needed for advancement.

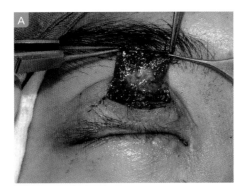 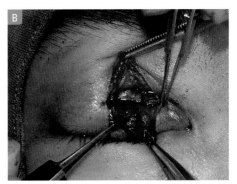

FIGURE 5-26 • **A.** The levator muscle is separated from conjunctiva. **B.** The separated levator muscle is advanced and fixed onto the tarsal plate.

Although resection of the horn requires greater amount of levator advancement, it also results in increased elasticity, which is helpful in reducing lid lag **(FIGURE 5-26A)**. However, the author finds that avoiding lateral horn exicision is usually the advantageous move.

Levator shortening

This technique is more appropriate for severe ptosis, which cannot be adequately addressed by methods mentioned above. The pretarsal tissue should be meticulously excised to secure the adhesion between advancement tissue and the tarsal plate. The levator muscle is advanced such that the upper eyelid margin rests on the upper limbus of cornea. The advanced portion of muscle is fixated with 6-0 nylon sutures at 3 points and additional 7-0 sutures inbetween. The fixation points are all located at 2 mm below the upper border of tarsal plate. The tarsal fixation should be placed securely, with partial thickness purchase into the cartilaginous substance, to avoid loosening of the levator complex from the tarsal structure. If the tarsal plate is weak or too thin, the suture needle can be driven twice through the plate to increase the fixation strength. If the free end of the levator muscle is short, it can be left alone. If it is too long, the extra bulk can become a cause for pretarsal fullness. In the latter situation, the extra tissue should be trimmed **(FIGURE 5-26B)**.

The maximum levator resection is 25 mm, and the "super maximum" resection refers to any advancement close to 30 mm. The levator muscle will retain its elasticity only to a certain degree of advancement. Beyond this point, elasticity of the

WAIT A MINUTE!

1. The dissection between levator muscle and conjunctiva may be impossible in patients with history of multiple operations. In such cases, a simpler solution is to treat the levator muscle and conjunctiva as a single layer and to resect the conjunctiva along with the levator. This does not lead to prolapse of the conjunctiva.

2. Depending on the surgeon, Müller's muscle is transected at upper border of the tarsal plate or a few millimeters above this border. At this point of the operation, the structure of the Müller's muscle is an important consideration. The Müller's muscle has a thickness of 0.7 ± 0.5 mm proximally and becomes thinner in the inferior portion. At 2 mm above upper border of tarsal plate, much of the muscle is replaced with a trabecular of connective tissue, which connects the muscle to the tarsal plate. This is sometimes referred to as the tendon of Müller's muscle. This tendon is reported to have a length of 2.56 mm (1.40-5.64 mm) and a thickness of 0.27 mm (0.08-0.88 mm). Transection of the muscle at about 1 mm above the tarsal border can provide a cleaner edge. Any resection above few millimeters would result in an uneven edge and make for a difficult advancement **(FIGURE 5-27)**.

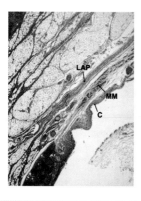

FIGURE 5-27 • Histology of the Müller's muscle.
The muscle (MM) consists of several bundles of smooth muscle and is located between levator aponeurosis (LAP) and conjunctiva (C). The Müller's muscle is connected to the tarsal plate (Ta) by a fibrous connective tissue (Müller's tendon, MT). Superiorly, there is a potential space between the aponeurosis and the muscle (post-aponeurotic space). Closer towards the tarsal plate, however, this space is obliterated by connective tissue. Because of this, the dissection is easier superiorly and more difficult inferiorly. Müller's muscle is thicker proximally and becomes thinner as it approaches the tarsal plate.

muscle decreases significantly, which can lead to lagophthalmos. This is related to the issue of exponential increase in tension versus length **(FIGURE 5-28)**. Because of this limitation, frontalis transfer or sling is indicated in ptosis with levator function less than 4 mm. However, some have argued for levator shortening even in the most severe forms of blepharoptosis. Berke et al. argued that levator shortening is more physiologic and is superior in both aesthetics and function to frontalis transfer. Mauriello reported satisfactory results after levator shortening in 28 out of 32 patients who had severe ptosis (> 4 mm) and poor levator function (< 2 mm). The disadvantage of levator shortening is that it is a more technically challenging operation, relative to frontalis operation **(FIGURE 5-29)**.

FIGURE 5-28 •

Relation of muscle elongation and stress.

The stress increases as the length of muscle increases. The relationship is linear at relatively lower muscle length but becomes exponential at greater lengths.

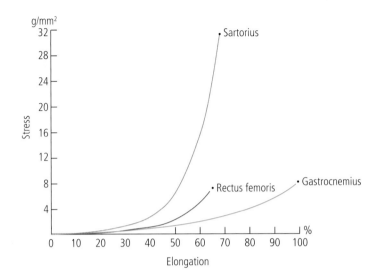

👆 **WAIT A MINUTE!**

PTOSIS RECURRENCE & LAGOPHTHALMOS

Ultimately, the two major problems with correction of severe ptosis is that, first, ptosis recurrence is an issue and that the recurrence occurs to an unpredictable degree and that, second, patients develop lagophthalmos with subsequent risk for exposure keratitis and other ophthalmologic complications. When considering the choice of operation, the surgeon must keep in mind these two problems and identify the operation with the least amount of risk for these postoperative complications. Correction of a severe ptosis to the same degree will result in different degrees of nocturnal lagophthalmos. The unfortunate fact of matter is that the author too frequently comes across patients who ended up with lagophthalmos despite initially having had relatively mild ptosis. At times, lagophthalmos may be an inevitable consequence of correcting a severe ptosis. However, a surgeon must do all that is within his ability to minimize this trade of one disability for another.

The reason some patients end up with significantly worse lagophthalmos is as follows:

1. The orbicularis oculi muscle is weak. Some patients with ptosis have weak orbicularis oculi muscle and suffer from nocturnal lagophthalmos while never having had any eyelid operation. This is because the levator muscle has undergone fibrosis and lost the elasticity. In patients with prior operation, the excision of pretarsal orbicularis muscle can contribute to the lagophthalmos. Therefore, it is highly important that pretarsal orbicularis muscle should not be excised at any cost.

2. The levator aponeurosis is significantly less elastic than Müller's muscle. Because of this, it is better to advance the Müller muscle to a greater degree than aponeurosis during Müller plicaiton.

3. In a previous ptosis operation, the levator muscle was advanced together with an inelastic structure such as the septum. The levator complex must be free from adjacent structures.

4. Iatrogenic trauma to the levator muscle can decrease the elasticity by fibrotic change.

5. Levator shortening requires full thickness resection of the muscle. A partial thickness excision of the levator muscle can result in suboptimal correction of the ptosis all the while worsening the lagophthalmos.

6. It is better to advance multiple tissues in small increments than to advance a single layer to an extreme degree, to obtain the same level of ptosis correction. For example, it is better to combine levator shortening and check ligament operation than to use levator shortening alone.

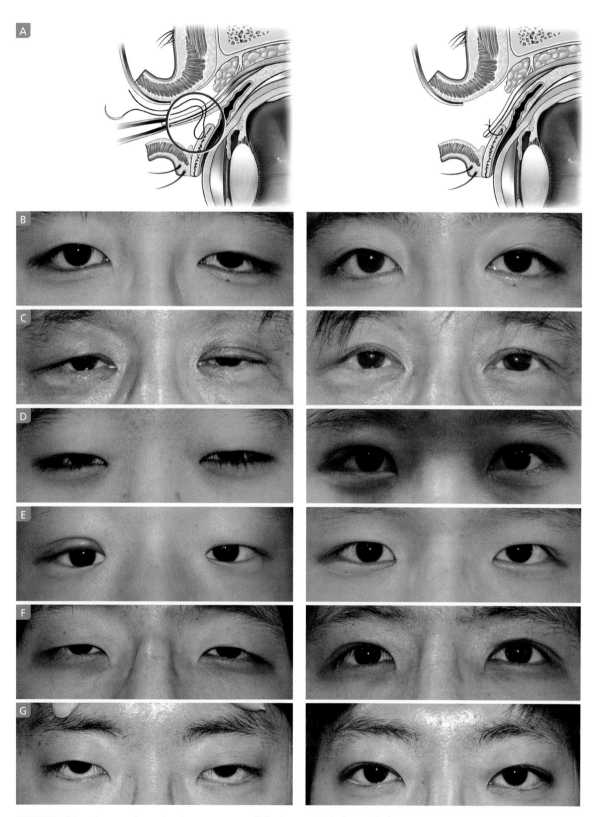

FIGURE 5-29 • Levator shortening in severe cases of blepharoptosis. Before and after surgery.

WAIT A MINUTE!

WHY IS UNDER-THROUGH LEVATOR PLICATION AVOIDED FOR SEVERE BLEPHAROPTOSIS?

Because of the mass effect. Levator shortening method has minimal mass effect, but the plication method results in greater mass effect with greater degree of tissue plication. Also, plication results in less secure adhesion than levator shortening.

Eyelid crease

- To create the eyelid crease, orbicularis oculi is fixated onto the tarsal plate. The eyelid crease forms relatively easily in the central and medial portions of the eyelid, because levator is advanced in central and medial portion. However, the levator muscle is not advanced in the lateral portion of the eyelid, and the eyelid crease can become faint or disappear. Also, it's easy for the eyelid crease to be higher in the lateral aspect. Generally, ptosis correction does not effect the lateral portion of the eyelid. To create a defined crease, the orbicularis muscle should be fixated not only to the tarsal plate but also to the aponeurosis at a higher location – to prevent the tarsal fixation from becoming undone. If the ptosis correction is performed to the central portion of the eyelid, the medial tarsal plate should be fixed to the aponeurosis as well.

- The skin is closed.

- If corneal exposure is severe, the lower eyelid can be brought up to cover the cornea with a Frost suture. This protects the cornea and also prevents potential stretching of the upper eyelid fixture from forcible closing of the eyelids.

The disadvantage of levator muscle shortening is that tissue trauma is significant. The separation of the muscle from the conjunctiva requires quite a bit of anesthetics, which can cause changes to the muscular function. The advantage of levator shortening is that it can be used in severe cases of ptosis and that recurrence of ptosis is less frequent because the advancement is more secure. The author usually employs levator shortening for ptosis greater than 2 mm. The technique can be used for milder forms of ptosis (less than 2 mm), but simpler methods of correction, such as the under-through technique, is much more appropriate. Even in mild ptosis, levator shortening method is indicated for severe scarring of the levator muscle from a previous operation.

Indication

- Moderate-to-severe ptosis
- Mild ptosis with prior operation and tissue scarring

Comparisons between various levator operations

A. Aponeurosis advancement: This technique is most frequently used for acquired or aponeurotic ptosis. It has been used for congenital cases, but this is associated with high rates of recurrence.

B. Müller plication and aponeurosis advancement: This combination is associated with lower rates of recurrence than either of the techniques alone. This can be used for both congenital and acquired forms of ptosis but is associated with high rates of recurrence in reoperative cases.

C. Under-through levator complex plication: This technique is associated with lower recurrence rate, compared with either aponeurosis advance or Müller plication. The mass effect in this method is similar to that of the plication-advancement complication.

D. Levator shortening: This method has the lowest rate of ptosis recurrence. It is applicable for severe ptosis.

The levator shortening operation has a major difference from other types of ptosis correction. During the operation, the levator muscle is completely disconnected from the tarsal plate, whereas the levator function is maintained in other techniques. During the operation, the levator function can be altered by anesthetics or by edema, which can be evaluated by undoing the plication suture. However, levator shortening does not allow this intraoperative evaluation of ptosis because the Müller muscle is separated from the tarsal plate, and there is no easy method of evaluating such changes except by placing fixation sutures.

Combination of levator shortening and under-through plication technique

Plication only is associated with ptosis recurrence in mild ptosis with prior history of operations and severe scarring. Such mild ptosis, however, does not always warrant levator shortening technique. In such cases, only the Müller's muscle can be dissected away from the conjunctiva above the tarsal plate with the rest of the complex plicated. This results in a more secure ptosis repair.

Prolapse of conjunctiva

After a wide dissection of the levator muscle from the conjunctiva, shortening the levator muscle by more than 15 mm will result in redundancy of the conjunctiva, which is a cause for prolapse. In milder cases, the prolapse may resolve spontaneously once the edema subsides and the conjunctiva contracts. Persistent prolapse is not only a problem aesthetically, but prolonged pressure can cause corneal ulcer.

To prevent this complication, the conjunctiva near the fornix can be sutured and stabilized with a bolster suture brought outside the eyelid skin **(FIGURE 5-30A)**. The bolster suture should be loose enough to allow free movement of the levator muscle. An alternative to the bolster suture is the fixation of the fornix conjunctiva to the aponeurosis. This latter method is more definitive than the pullout bolster suture **(FIGURE 5-30B)**.

Injection of hyaluronidase can be helpful in reducing the prolapsed conjunctiva. If the levator advancement is great, the conjunctiva must also be shortened. The edges of the conjunctiva should be approximated accurately and securely to avoid the formation of mucoid cyst. In practice, the author first attempts bolster suture method on any suspected prolapse. If this is not sufficient in preventing the formation of prolapse, the prolapsed portion of the conjunctiva is excised, with resultant

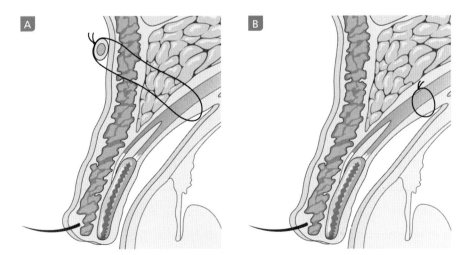

FIGURE 5-30 • Treatment of conjunctival prolapse.
A. pull-out suture of conjunctiva. **B.** Fixation through the levator muscle onto the aponeurosis.

edges coming together without much tension. If the prolapse is discovered several days after the surgery, the adhesion of the conjunctiva does not allow the suture technique, and it is better to directly excise the exposed conjunctiva after topical anesthesia. Besides the pullout bolster suture, another suture technique involves the fixation of the fornix conjunctiva to just the aponeurosis. This method is more definitive than the pullout bolster suture method **(FIGURE 5-31)**.

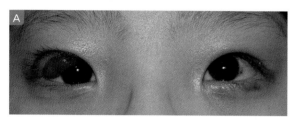 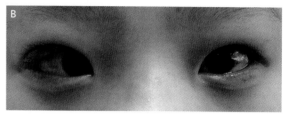

FIGURE 5-31 • Conjunctival prolapse and correction.

TABLE 5-2 • The differences between levator plication techniques and levator shortening techniques.

	Levator complex plication (under-through technique)	Levator shortening
Applicable degree of ptosis	Mild-to-moderate ptosis	Moderate-to-severe ptosis
Degree of surgical trauma	Mild	Moderate
Intraoperative levator examination	Possible	Not possible
Sensitivity to local anesthetic	Sensitive	Occasional
Conjunctival prolapse	No	Occasional
Recurrence rate	Occasional	Rare

The difference between levator complex plication and levator shortening. *Unlike levator shortening, levator plication leaves the Müller's muscle attached to the tarsal plate.

 WAIT A MINUTE!

WHY ARE PLICATION TECHNIQUES SUCH AS THE UNDER-THROUGH TECHNIQUE NOT USED FOR SEVERE PTOSIS?

Because of mass effect. In plication techniques, the advancement of levator complex may meet a significant amount of resistance around the upper border of tarsal plate. Advancements under 10 mm is not a big problem, but advancements greater than that amount does not yield any significant gain.

Check ligament and conjoined fascial sheath operation

In the history of ptosis surgery, the use of check ligament represents a significant innovation after a relatively stagnant period of incremental changes. In 2002, Holmström introduced a new method of correcting ptosis, by the fixation of check ligament of the superior fornix of conjunctival sac to the tarsal plate. The structure is referred by various terms, but the author prefers the term "check ligament" as it was originally called by Holmström and the term "conjoined fascial sheath (CFS)" as an anatomically descriptive name. Hwang et al. have expounded on the anatomy and operative methods for CFS. In severe ptosis, the author advances the CFS suspension and the levator muscle simultaneously. This combined approach distributes the weight of eyelid to the levator muscle and the CFS, which increases the elasticity of the structure and decreases the risk of lagophthalmos. This is because the elasticity of the ligament and levator muscle decreases significantly with stretching (FIGURE 5-32).

Check ligament (CFS)

The check ligament is a plate of connective tissues, which connects with 1) the sheath of levator muscle, 2) the sheath of superior rectus muscle, and 3) Tenon's capsule. The ligament serves to stabilize the superior fornix (FIGURE 5-33). Around the fornix, the ligament is 2 mm long around the bulbar conjunctiva and palpebral conjunctiva, and this proportion of the check ligament is aptly called "conjunctival extension". More proximally to this, the ligament extends about 15 mm between the levator muscle and superior rectus muscle. The structure is a highly elastic

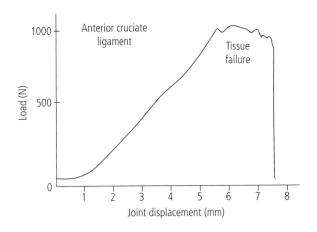

FIGURE 5-32 •
Relationship between load and joint displacement.

connective tissue. In ptosis correction, advancement of the check ligament results in elevation of the eyelid with upward gaze because of the superior rectus muscle is coupled to the levator mechanism. Because of the high elasticity of the resulting mechanism, lagophthalmos occurs with less frequency, compared to other operations. The ligament can be advanced to the most proximal portion to the most distal portion (conjunctival extension) according to the severity of ptosis **(FIGURE 5-34)**.

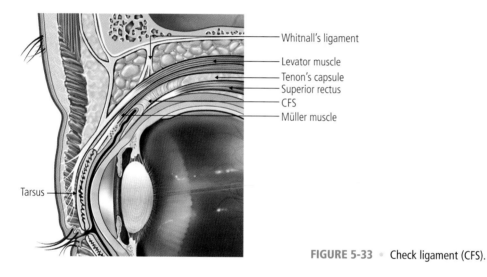

FIGURE 5-33 ● Check ligament (CFS).

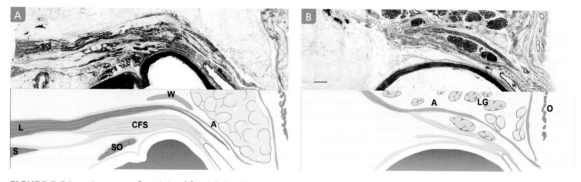

FIGURE 5-34 ● Anatomy of conjoined fascial sheath. Microscopic findings and illustrations.
A. sagittal cross-section through midpupillary line. **B.** cross-section through lateral limbus line.
Conjoined fascial sheath (CFS) is located in the intermuscular space between the anterior one third of superior rectus muscle (S) and segment of levator muscle (L). Posteriorly, it was extended from the fascia of the levator and superior rectus. Anteriorly, superficial and deep extensions (arrows) of CFS are continued about 2 mm to the superior conjunctival fornix, then 2-3 mm distally (arrow heads) along and beneath the palpebral and bulbar conjunctiva. W: Whitnall's superior transverse ligament, A: levator aponeurosis, SO: superior oblique muscle, F: preaponeurotic fat, OS: orbital septum, O: orbicularis oculi muscle, LG: lacrimal gland. (Histology reprinted with permission from Hwang)

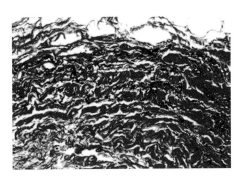

FIGURE 5-35 • Histology of check ligament.
Red: collagen fiber. Blue: elastic fiber. (From reference 15)

Histology of check ligament

The ligament is composed of collagen and elastic fibers. Because of the elastic fibers, check ligament is a highly elastic structure. It does not contain any muscle cells (FIGURE 5-35).

The author's technique

Check ligament (CFS) suspension combined with levator shortening

Local anesthesia

This technique is used for severe ptosis, and the levator function is limited. Because of this, the anesthetic solution does not affect the eyelid position as much, and liberal application of anesthetic containing epinephrine is recommended.

Skin incision and dissection

The skin incision is made along the eyelid crease to be made. The orbicularis muscle and orbital septum are divided to expose the levator aponeurosis. The pretarsal tissue is excised enough to expose the tarsal plate. If the tarsal plate is not exposed adequately, the adhesion may not be enough, which can become a cause for ptosis recurrence.

The space between conjunctiva and Müller's muscle is hydro-dissected with a 1:3 dilution of a mixture containing 2% lidocaine and 1:100,000 epinephrine with saline.

The incision is placed while being careful to protect the peripheral arterial arcade, and the dissection is carried between the Müller's muscle and conjunctiva. This step

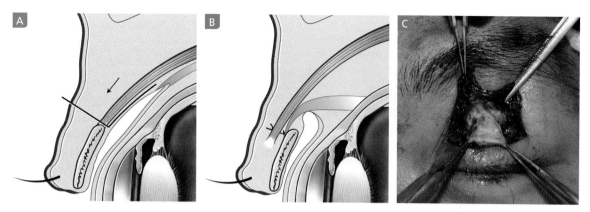

FIGURE 5-36 • **A.** The dissection is carried between the levator muscle and the conjunctiva. **B.** Both the levator muscle and CFS are advanced and fixated onto the tarsal plate. **C.** The levator muscle is held in the forceps by the eyebrow. The CFS is held by the two pairs of forceps close to the eyelid margin.

is similar to the dissection in levator shortening. Blunt dissection in the superior direction will reveal a smooth, thick, opaque, and glistening membrane at the fornix level, which is the check ligament (CFS). This ligament is advanced and fixated with 6-0 nylon. The height of eyelid is adjusted by the location of fixation (proximal or distal) on the check ligament.

The check ligament is elastic in its distal portion near the fornix, but this elasticity decreases in proximally. To a certain degree of advancement, the risk of lagophthalmos is low, but the elasticity decreases abruptly at a superior point, beyond which lagophthalmos becomes a significant problem **(FIGURE 5-31)**. This decrease in elasticity is the limiting factor for how much ptosis can be corrected by check ligament advancement. The author uses as much of the elasticity provided by the check ligament and the remaining degree of ptosis is corrected by the advancement in levator muscle. Similarly, the levator muscle also has a similar length-elasticity relationship. By dividing the job of advancement between the levator muscle and the check ligament, most severe cases of ptosis can be addressed without causing lagophthalmos **(FIGURE 5-36)**. Usually, the author determines the proportion of ptosis to be advanced first using the check ligament and the remainder of advancement is made using the levator muscle. The evaluation of eyelid height is best evaluated in the sitting position.

This combined operation is employed for severe cases of ptosis. The operation should anticipate and overcorrect for 2 mm of postoperative depression.

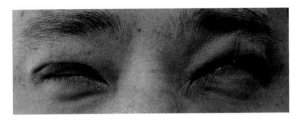

FIGURE 5-37 • Frost suture on left lower lid.

Eyelid crease

Upon correction of ptosis, the eyelid crease is created by the fixation of orbicularis oculi muscle to the tarsal plate using a 7-0 PDS.

The lateral portion of the eyelid is not involved in the ptosis correction process. Because of this, the eyelid crease is higher laterally and can become faint over time. To avoid this, the orbicularis muscle close to the skin incision should be fixated to the tarsal plate and to the aponeurosis 5 mm above the tarsal plate. (3-point fixation)

The skin is closed. For severe cases of ptosis, the skin edged should be everted to avoid scar depression.

Frost suture is placed in preparation for nocturnal lagophthalmos (FIGURE 5-37).

Another advantage of this operation is that the advancement of check ligament leads to advancement of the fornix, which decreases the risk of conjunctival prolapse (FIGURE 5-38).

Frontalis muscle transfer

- Frontalis muscle flap transfer
- Frontalis myofascial flap transfer
- Frontalis sling operation

This technique is useful for patients with severe ptosis without any levator function but who are able to create forehead creases using the frontalis muscle. The first such operation using frontalis muscle to elevate the upper eyelid was reported by Fergus in 1901. This technique was subsequently improved on and reported by Song and Song in 1982. To increase the range of advancement, Zhou and Chang introduced the frontalis myofascial flap transfer in 1988.

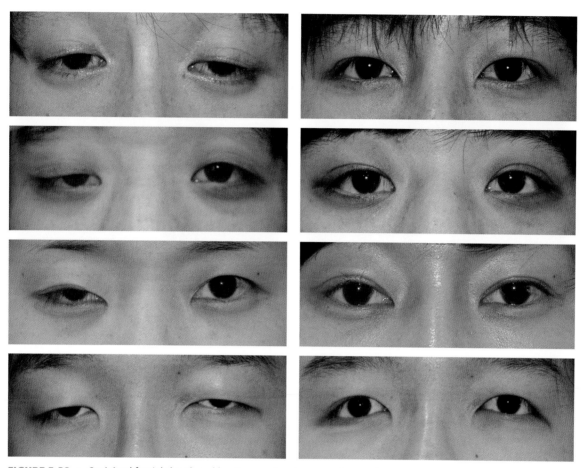

FIGURE 5-38 • Conjoined fascial sheath and levator muscle advancement operation.

Of the three techniques, the author prefers flap transfers to the sling operation because of the directness and the lack of need for a separate donor site. Between the two flap transfers, the myofascial transfer is more robust and allows for more advancement, which translates into requiring smaller back-cuts The problems of the frontalis operations are that it is difficult to obtain symmetrical palpebral fissure and that the operation leaves scars in the forehead (and in the thigh for the sling operation). The risk for ptosis recurrence is always present.

The frontalis myofascial flap transfer will be discussed here.

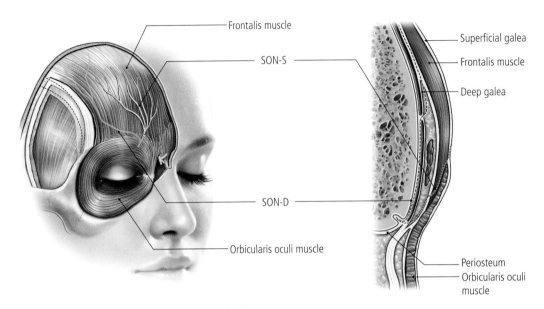

FIGURE 5-39 • Anatomic course of the supraorbital nerve.
SON-S – superficial branches of the nerve. SON-D – deep branches.

Frontalis myofascial flap transfer

Operative details

Design

After designing the eyelid crease and marking the supraorbital notch, a 1.5 cm horizontal incision is designed lateral to the notch to avoid the injury to the supraorbital nerve bundle.

Elevation of the frontalis myofascial flap

Upon local anesthesia, the eyelid skin is incised. The dissection is carried past the orbicularis muscle, exposing the tarsal plate. The 1.5 cm subbrow incision is made, and subcutaneous dissection is carried down to the frontalis muscle. At the superior orbital rim, the lowermost portion of frontalis fascia is opened 2-to-2.5 cm horizontally. The frontalis myofascial flap is dissected superficially between the frontalis muscle and skin and deeply between the frontal periosteum and the galea. At this point, it is important to protect the deep branch of the supraorbital nerve. At times, the dissection maybe omitted for the deep plane. Additionally, care must

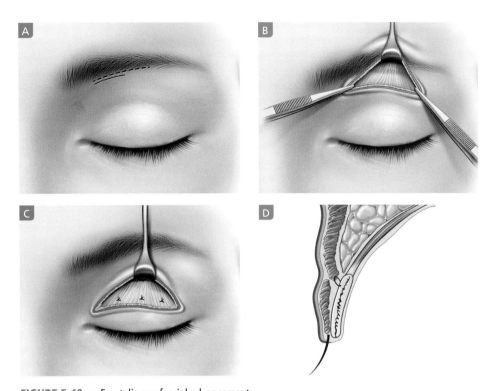

FIGURE 5-40 • Frontalis myofascial advancement.
A. A 1.5-cm subbrow incision and the eyelid crease incision. **B.** The frontalis muscle is exposed deep to the eyebrow.
C, D. Through the blepharoplasty incision, the advanced frontalis muscle is secured to the tarsal plate.

be taken not to injure the temporal branch of facial nerve. The deep branch of supraorbital nerve exits the supraorbital notch and travels superolaterally between the periosteum and galea and exits superficially through the galea about 3 cm above the supraorbital notch. The superficial branch stays superficial to the frontalis muscle from the notch **(FIGURE 5-39)**.

Laterally to the supraorbital nerve a 1-cm back-cut is made on the frontalis muscle, and the flap is elevated **(FIGURE 5-40)**.

Frontalis myofascial flap transfer

The tunnel is created between orbicularis muscle and orbital septum, which is not wider than the muscle flap. The flap is brought down through the tunnel and fixated to the tarsal plate such that the eyelid margin rests on the upper corneal limbus, which represents a 2 mm of overcorrection.

Eyelid crease operation

The crease is made by the fixation of orbicularis muscle to the advanced frontalis aponeurosis. Laterally, the eyelid crease does not form easily. A 3-point fixation is helpful in securing the eyelid crease (tarsal plate, frontalis muscle fascia, and orbicularis muscle). The skin is closed, and compression bandage is applied to the forehead.

The advantage in frontalis transfer over levator advancement is in postoperative lagophthalmos. In severe cases of ptosis, levator advancement can result in lagophthalmos even if the advancement is conservative. However, conservative frontalis advancement does not necessarily cause lagophthalmos. Thus, patients who benefit

---

WAIT A MINUTE!

The advancement required to fixate the frontalis fascia to the tarsal plate is not as much as it is commonly believed. The flap is fixated 2 mm below the upper border of tarsal plate while the eyelids are open. The frontalis is fixated at about a height that is 15 mm superior to the lower eyelid margin, which means a centimeter of advancement is more than adequate and not a whole lot of frontalis muscle needs to be dissected nor is a big back-cut required. This obviates the need for additional techniques or materials for extending the frontalis muscle such as frontalis-orbicularis flap **(FIGURE 5-41, 5-42)**.

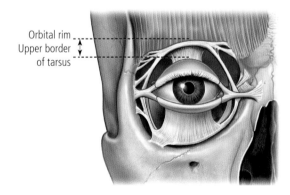

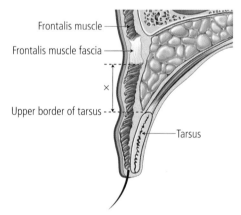

FIGURE 5-41 • The distance between tarsal plate and orbital rim.
With the eyelids open, the upper border of tarsal plate is less than 5 mm away from the orbital rim.

FIGURE 5-42 • The distance between frontalis fascia and tarsal plate.
The fascia (or tendon) of frontalis muscle inserts into the orbital rim. The muscle is advanced to the tarsal plate while the eyes are open, and the distance between the fascia and the upper border of tarsal plate is less than 10 mm.

the most from frontalis transfer are those who have low tolerance against lagoph-thalmos – oculomotor nerve palsy, Bell's phenomenon, history of corneal operation, etc. – but have decent frontalis muscle activity.

The disadvantage of this method is asymmetry of the eyebrow and forehead creases in patients with unilateral ptosis **(FIGURE 5-43)**.

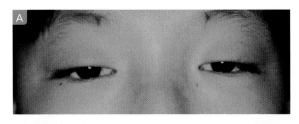
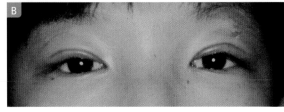
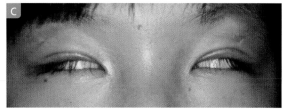

FIGURE 5-43 • Photographs before and after frontalis transfer.

 WAIT A MINUTE!

Several variables must be considered when frontalis transfer is used to correct ptosis. Slight loss of eyelid height is always inevitable. The loss of eyelid height is dependent on the robustness of the surgical construct and the fixations. Another consideration is to decrease the amount of advancement in patients who use the frontalis muscle frequently, which decreases the risk of lagophthalmos. Also, the eyelid height should be adjusted according to the corneal resistance to exposure keratitis for each patient.

OTHER TYPES OF BLEPHAROPTOSIS

Jaw-winking ptosis (Marcus-Gunn syndrome)

Jaw-winking ptosis is caused by misdirection of the trigeminal nerve (CN V) signal to the oculomotor nerve (CN III). In this syndrome, activation of the jaw muscle is accompanied by simultaneous activation of the contralateral levator palpebrae superioris muscle. Opening, closing, or side movement of the lower jaw will elicit raising of the ptotic eyelid. Jaw-winking ptosis represents 4-to-6% of all congenital ptosis and is usually unilateral with preponderance for the left side.

Operative details

The two main variables to consider are the degree of ptosis and the amount of eyelid elevation with jaw movement.

The ptosis correction should preserve as much of the levator function as possible, if the ptosis is mild or if the eyelid elevation is mild with jaw movement. However, if the levator dysfunction is severe, the muscle should be resected completely, and the eyelid should be controlled by either the frontalis muscle or by the superior rectus muscle via check ligament. This synkinetic movement has been known to resolve spontaneously over time.

Horner's syndrome

The ptosis of Horner's syndrome is caused by a defect in the sympathetic trunk leading to paralysis of the Müller's muscle, and can be congenital or acquired in nature.

Main symptoms

- The degree of ptosis coincides with the range of motion for Müller's muscle (2-3 mm). The ipsilateral lower eyelid is slightly elevated.
- Miosis
- Enophthalmos
- Depigmentation of the iris (FIGURE 5-44A)
- Anhydrosis of the ipsilateral face and neck

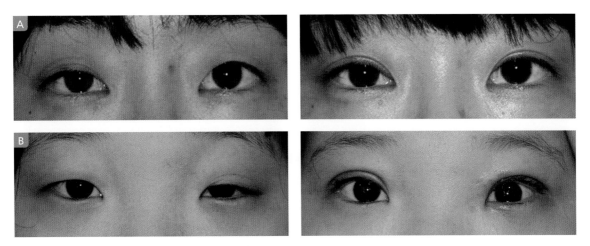

FIGURE 5-44 • Operative correction of Horner syndrome.
A. This patient has right-sided ptosis, miosis, and iris depigmentation. **B.** In this patient, the upper eyelid ptosis is accompanied with eyelvated lower eyelid margin.

Horner's syndrome can be caused by any number of pathologic entities along the sympathetic chain. Main causes are tumor, infection, aneurysm, head trauma, and iatrogenic trauma. In certain cases, treatment of the primary cause can lead to restoration of function (i.e. releasing compressive tumor). Otherwise, the ptosis itself can be corrected using ptosis correction techniques.

The ptosis of Horner's syndrome is caused by the paralysis of Müller's muscle. However, the syndrome is caused by a preganglionic lesion, and unlike postganglionic problems, the myoneural junction remains intact. As such, the application of epinephrine or phenylephrine will result in pupillary dilation and eyelid elevation. Because the Müller's muscle has not been under innervation, the eyelid may rise above the height of the contralateral eye. 1) Small amount of epinephrine may lead to 3 mm of eyelid elevation, which can be lead to undercorrection of ptosis. 2) The pupil is smaller than normal, and this can lead to apparent decrease in eyelid height on the involved side. 3) The lower eyelid margin is higher than the contralateral side, and thus the palpebral fissure will still be smaller even if the upper eyelid margins are at the same height. 4) For another yet-unknown reason, the palpebral fissure decreases in the postoperative period. For these reasons, ptosis of Horner's syndrome requires overcorrection, unequivocally. Because the Müller's muscle is extra sensitive to epinephrine, the use of epinephrine should be minimized as much as possible. The degree of ptosis will most likely be around 2 mm. As such, techniques for mild-to-moderate ptosis are appropriate (i.e. levator shortening and under-through levator plication).

RECURRENCE OF PTOSIS

The rate of recurrence varies according to patient factors, choice of operation, and the surgeon's technique. Severity of the ptosis correlates with the amount of recurrence. Secure correction of ptosis tends to decrease the risk of recurrence.

The levator complex operations can be used as an example. In the author's experience, recurrence is highest for aponeurotic surgery, followed in the decreasing order by Müller tuck and aponeurosis advancement, levator complex plication, and levator resection. Compared to CFS advancement alone, the combination of CFS advancement and levator shortening results in a much more secure surgical construct, which decreases the rate of recurrence.

Even for the same operation, the recurrence rate might be affected by minor technical differences. For example, higher number of advancement sutures decreases the recurrence of ptosis. The author places 3 sutures for mild cases of ptosis but places 5 sutures for moderate-to-severe ptosis. Also, the proper excision of pretarsal soft tissue is important for provide a secure adhesion between the advanced tissue and tarsal plate.

Recurrence rate can vary by the etiology behind ptosis. Recurrence rate is lower for aponeurotic ptosis than for congenital ptosis. The author does not use levator aponeurosis advancement for congenital potsis because of higher recurrence rate and reserves the operation for aponeurotic ptosis.

For example, dehisced aponeurosis requires 1-to-1.5 mm of overcorrection for aponeurosis advancement (Anderson). Because of this requirement for overcorrection, the addition of Müller plication to aponeurosis advancement is helpful in reducing ptosis recurrence.

UNILATERAL PTOSIS AND ASYMMETRIC PTOSIS

For unilateral ptosis, it is important to minimize the potential effect of anesthestics and edema has on the eyelid position. If the eyelid position does change, however, it is important to note the degree of change in the eyelid height and to account for this change when correcting the ptosis. For instance, if the anesthesia resulted in a 1 mm decrease in the eyelid position, then the operation should incorporate a 1-mm undercorrection to account for increase in eyelid height once the anesthesia wears off.

During the operation for unilateral ptosis, the eyelid position should be compared while evaluating whether the non-ptotic eyelid remains the usual position. The goal of ptosis correction is to obtain symmetric eyelid heights with primary gaze, provided that the ptotic eyelid will be lower with wide-open eyes and will be higher with slightly open eyelids. Before the operation, a patient with unilateral ptosis should be examined for how much of the eyelid height may change, according to Hering's law. If the patient opens the non-ptotic eye to a lesser degree than usual, the ptotic eyelid will be undercorrected. The non-ptotic eye will exhibit Hering's Law to a greater degree if the ptotic eyelid is over the dominant eye.

In highly asymmetric ptosis, recurrence is more likely on the side with severe ptosis. For example, the eyelid with mild ptosis is overcorrected by 0.5-to-1 mm whereas the side with severe ptosis is overcorrected by 2 mm, for a difference of 1-to-1.5 mm in overcorrection between the eyes (FIGURES 5-45, 5-46, 5-48).

Asymmetric ptosis

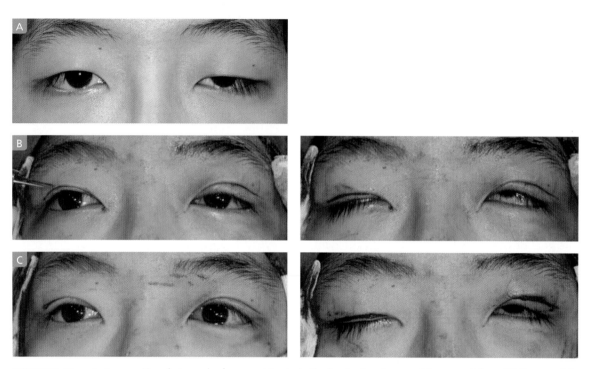

FIGURE 5-45 ● **A.** Preoperative photograph of asymmetric ptosis. The levator function was 10 mm on right and 5-6 mm on left. **B.** Intraoperative photograph. Right eyelid was elevated with Müller tuck and aponeurosis advancement. Left eyelid was elevated with check ligament advancement only, which was not adequate. Left photograph is eyes open in sitting position. Right photograph is of the patient with closed eyes. Lagophthalmos is significant on the left eye. **C.** The levator muscle was shortened in the left eyelid. The advancement was performed in a 4:1 ratio between check ligament advancement and levator shortening. The left palpebral fissure is taller than right.

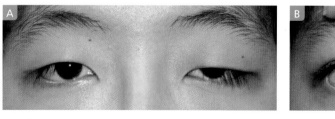

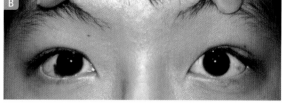

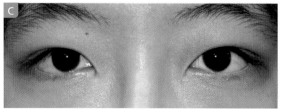

FIGURE 5-46 ● Pre/postoperative photograph of the patient from **FIGURE 5-45**.

The left eyelid had been overcorrected by 1.5 mm, which was the more severely ptotic side. **A.** Preoperative photograph. **B.** At 2 weeks after operation, the left eyelid is slightly higher. **C.** At 15 months after operation, the eyelid margins are at the same height.

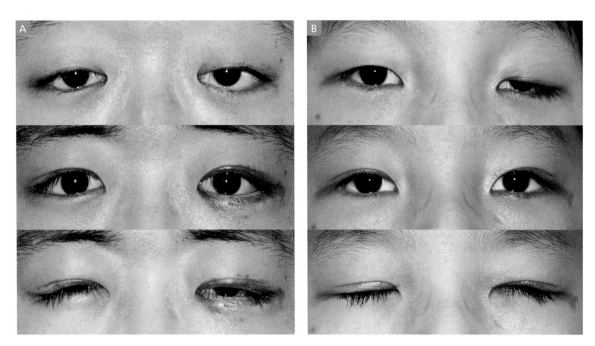

FIGURE 5-47 • Comparison of bilateral and unilateral ptosis.
A. Bilateral ptosis. **B.** Unilateral ptosis.
Top: Preoperative photographs. Middle: Postoperative photographs with eyes open. Bottom: Postoperative photographs with eyes closed.
In the patient with unilateral ptosis (**B**), the ptotic left eyelid has greater degree of lagophthalmos after the operation.

PARTIALLY PTOTIC EYELIDS

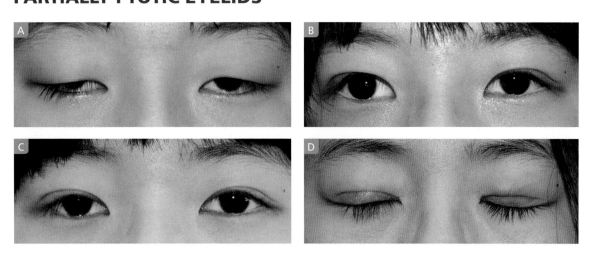

FIGURE 5-48 • Asymmetric ptosis.
A. The ptosis is more severe on the right side. **B.** At 2 weeks after operation, the right eyelid demonstrates overcorrection. **C.** At 15 months, the eyelid height is similar between both eyes. **D.** The right side shows a slight lagophthalmos, as expected from the preoperative difference in ptosis severity.

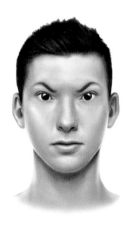

FIGURE 5-49 • Persons with medial ptosis are portrayed as sly or deceitful.

Medial or lateral ptosis

Ptosis can be partially severe in the medial or lateral portion of the eyelid. Medial ptosis can give off a sly or deceitful intent **(FIGURE 5-49)**, whereas lateral ptosis can be misconstrued as a lazy or lethargic characteristic of the person.

The logically simple solution to this is to partially correct the ptosis where it is most prominent. One important consideration to this solution is that the partial advancement must overcorrect the portion of involved eyelid. For medial ptosis, the overcorrection will result in laterally dropping palpebral fissure in the immediate postoperative period. Another important point is that partial corrections should incorporate adjacent or central portion of the eyelid because the levator apparatus is wide.

Medial ptosis tends to recur frequently because of anatomic characteristics specific to the medial eyelid. A wide area of the medial eyelid is devoid of any levator muscle, which is larger than the levator-less area in the lateral eyelid. This medial area is called a "bare area". Fixation of the connective tissue to tarsal plate in this bare area can result in temporary elevation of eyelid, which will gradually become ptotic again **(FIGURE 5-50B)**.

THE DIFFICULTY IN ACCURATE CORRECTION OF PTOSIS

In ptosis correction, fixed advancement of tissue does not result in consistent degree of ptosis correction. The eyelid height is known to change with general anesthesia (Brown), as well as for local anesthesia. A number of factors influence the eyelid height.

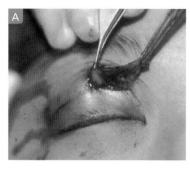
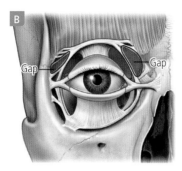
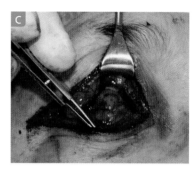

FIGURE 5-50 • **A.** Partial advancement of the medial levator muscle. **B.** Elevation of the medial eyelid is often ineffective because of the large gap in the levator structure. Laterally, this is less of a problem. **C.** The medial border of Müller's muscle is marked with ink. The gap adjustment to this margin is large. (Refer to **FIGURE 5-15**)

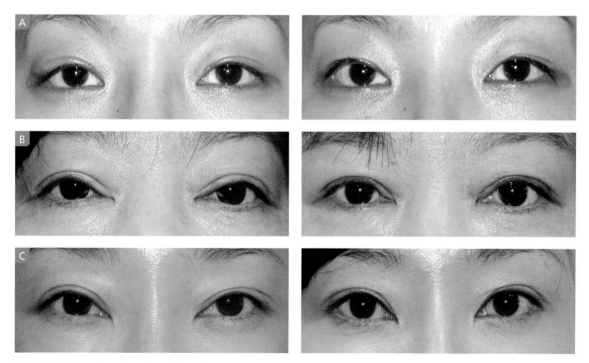

FIGURE 5-51 • Correction of medial ptosis.
A. Medial ptosis of right eye only. **B, C.** Medial ptosis in both eyes.

Intraoperative factors

- Local anesthetic, general anesthetic, or sedatives
- Edema or hematoma
- Position: recumbent versus sitting
- Hering's law: increased exposure to light in one eye affects the eyelid height of the other side
- Position of eyebrows
- Hyaluronidase
- Tarsal shift
- Vertical strabismus
- Excessive light exposure, patient anxiety
- Visual acuity, dominant eye
- Xerophthalmia
- Eyelid crease formation
- Release of adhesion

Postoperative factors

- Swelling
- Hematoma cheese wiring effect

Hering's law

Correction of unilateral ptosis can result in larger-than-intended palpebral fissure in the corrected eye and the development of ptosis in what used to be the normal eye. In 1977, Hering argued that this phenomenon arises from the fact that the both left and right eyelids are under the control of the same neural pathway. Correction of ptosis in one eye signals the brain to no longer sends out compensating motor signal to the frontalis and levator, which results in ptotic eyelid on what used to be the normal eye. Because of this, it is important to examine the normal-appearing eyelid for slight ptosis in a patient with asymmetric ptosis.

In many cases of unilateral ptosis, the degree of ptosis correction can sometimes be less than the actual difference between the heights of two eyelids. For a unilateral ptosis with 3 mm of eyelid height difference, the normal eyelid can settle down by about 0.5-to-1 mm after a unilateral ptosis correction. Therefore, the actual degree of ptosis correction needed is about 2-to-2.5 mm for a symmetrical height. This is especially the case if the unilateral ptosis is over the dominant eye (FIGURE 5-52F, G).

This phenomenon must be considered for bilateral ptosis as well. Correction of the ptosis over the first eye may appear too much, but the eyelid height can be

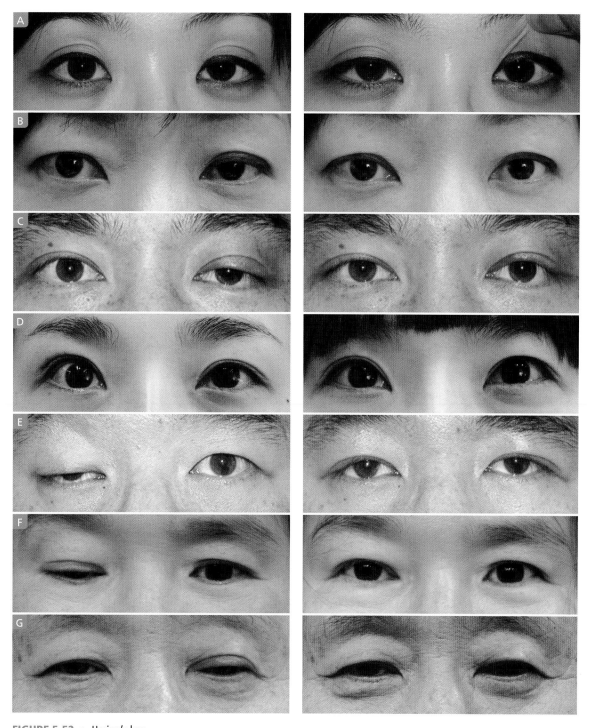

FIGURE 5-52 • Hering's law.

Hering's law positive. **A.** Manual elevation test. Lifting the ptotic left eyelid leads to a decrease in eyelid height on the contralateral side. **B.** Phenylephrine test. Left: Ptotic left eye. Right: Instillation of phenylephrine in the ptotic eye leads to elevation of the right eyelid. **C.** Correction of the left ptotic eyelid lowers the contralateral eyelid margin. **D.** Correction of right eyelid retraction is associated with elevation of the left eyelid. Hering's law negative **E.** Correction of ptosis on the right side lowers the left eyelid. **F.** In this patient with dominance in the left eye, correction of ptosis in the right eye does not lower the left eyelid. **G.** In this patient with dominance in the right eye, correction of left ptosis does not lower the right eye.

observed to decrease over the course of correcting the ptosis in the contralateral eye. Even if the eyelid that's operated first appears too high, the operator must resist the temptation to redo the fixation at a lower position. Instead, the contralateral eyelid should be elevated manually to see if the first eyelid adjusts to a more appropriate height.

Another corollary to this can be observed in the bilateral blepharoptosis, the frontalis and levator muscles are involuntarily contracted to allow light to enter through the pupils. However, correction of ptosis can remove this need to contract the frontalis and levator muscles, with involuntary drive gone. This is one significant reason why sometimes ptosis correction appears inadequate in the postoperative period despite intraoperative evaluation showing adequate correction. The author describes this as "laziness of eye opening muscles" to patients.

On physical exam, the Hering's law is considered positive if the decrease in contralateral eyelid height is greater than 1 mm. The examination is more frequently positive for acquired ptosis than for congenital ptosis and for patients whose dominant eye is affected by the ptosis.

According to reports, manual elevation test was positive in 10% to 29% among ptosis patients (Bodian, Tucker). Meyer reported manual elevation test to be positive in 20% of cases but the occlusion test to be positive in 4% of cases. The author is of the opinion that Hering's law is a lot more prevalent when considering the minute decreases in the eyelid height in the postoperative setting.

In contrast to ptosis, eyelid retraction can lead to decreased eyelid height in the contralateral side, and correction of the retraction can lead to increased eyelid height in the contralateral ptotic eye. Therefore, slight ptosis in one eye with retraction in the contralateral eye should not be corrected simultaneously. Rather, the surgeon must choose correcting either to ptosis or the retraction and observe postoperative changes in the contralateral eye.

Considerations in approaching concomitant ptosis and retraction

- Whether correction of the ptosis resolve the retraction in the contralateral eyelid
- Whether correction of the retraction resolve the ptosis in the contralateral eyelid
- Would both eyelids require correction?

Examinations for Hering's Law

1. Manual elevation test: The ptotic eyelid is elevated. The test is positive if the contralateral eyelid decreases in height.
2. Visual block test, eye occlusion test: The ptotic eye is blocked, and the contralateral eyelid is observed.
3. Sympathomimetic test: Phenylephrine is instilled in the ptotic eye. The contralateral eyelid is observed.

Effects of local anesthetic

Local anesthetics such as lidocaine and bupivacaine have the following effects:

1. Paralyses Müller's and levator muscles and decreases upper eyelid function.
2. Paralyses orbicularis muscle, which slightly elevates the upper eyelid.
3. The volume of injection causes edema, which decreases the ability to elevate the eyelid.
4. Epinephrine activates Müller's muscle and increases the eyelid height. The amount of elevation has been reported to be 1.0 mm after 10 minutes of epinephrine instillation (Bartley, 1995) and 1-to-1.5 mm (Brown).

These effects of local anesthetic are accentuated by the sensitiveness of muscle. In patients with mild ptosis (i.e. preserved levator function), the bare minimal of local anesthesia should be used. The inverse is also true; liberal use of anesthesia does not interfere with eyelid height in severe ptosis.

When the eyelid height changes due to local anesthesia, the operator must understand that this change will be temporary and that the ptosis correction must account for the cessation of this change after the operation. The same can be said for changes due to edema and hematoma.

Eyelid crease fixation

Fixation of eyelid crease can result in up to 1.5 mm decrease in palpebral fissure height. If the eyelid crease is asymmetric or unilateral, this variable must be addressed by performing the crease fixation before the correction of ptosis.

Eye dominance

Compared to non-dominant eye, the levator advancement may require less advancement in the dominant eye in proportion of cases.

PTOSIS CORRECTION WITH GENERAL ANESTHESIA

Unlike local anesthesia, general anesthesia does not allow for evaluation of eyelid height during the operation. The two method of ptosis correction under general anesthesia are 1) to decide preoperatively the amount of advancement, based on the severity of ptosis and levator function and 2) to adjust the eyelid height while under general anesthesia.

Determining the amount of advancement prior to operation

1. Like the method by Berke, congenital ptosis can be corrected by advancing the levator by 4 times the ptotic amount or by 2 times the ptotic amount plus 2 mm.
2. For aponeurotic ptosis, the tarso-aponeurectomy method can be used to advance the tissue by 3 mm plus ptotic amount (McCord), 2 mm plus ptotic amount (Chen), or to aponeuro-muscular junction (McCord).

Adjusting the eyelid height while under general anesthesia

Levator resection method

Levator function	Intraoperative eyelid height
5-6 mm	1-to-1.5 mm higher than desired position
7-8 mm	At desired position
9-10 mm	1 mm lower than desired position

Frontalis suspension

Levator function	Intraoperative eyelid height
0-2 mm	1 mm higher than desired position
3-4 mm	At desired position
5 mm	1 mm lower than desired position

☞ WAIT A MINUTE!

Between levator shortening and frontalis sling, the overlapping levator function is 5 mm. For levator shortening, the eyelid height is set at 1-to-1.5 mm higher than the desired position. For frontalis sling, the eyelid height is set at 1 mm lower than the desired position. Why is there a 2-to-2.5 mm difference between the two techniques if the levator function is the same? In both techniques, the eyelid height will become lower in the postoperative period, and overcorrection is necessary. However, one significant difference is in the frontalis muscle, which is usually contracted for ptosis patients but which is relaxed under general anesthesia. As such, frontalis sling requires under-correction.

POSTOPERATIVE OUTCOME AND MANAGEMENT

Intraoperative eyelid height can change from anesthetic or sedative agents, intraoperative edema, photosensitivity, patient anxiety, xerophthalmia, etc. In the postoperative period, the eyelid height can change from edema or loosening of the advanced tissue. Because of this, patients should be counseled on the potential need for adjustment of the ptosis correction at a later period.

No clear consensus exists on the appropriate time for a corrective operation. The author performs the corrective operation depending on the amount of edema. If the edema is minimal, a revision can be performed between days 3 and 5. If the edema is significant, the revision is performed between 7 and 12 days. However, if the edema or hematoma is excessive, the eyelid may rise in height with time. Additionally, intraoperative trauma to the levator muscle can allow for eyelid height elevation during the 6 months after operation. The eyelid height can also vary across different techniques. After Müller plication, the eyelid margin tends to come to a stable position relatively early in the postoperative period, whereas the

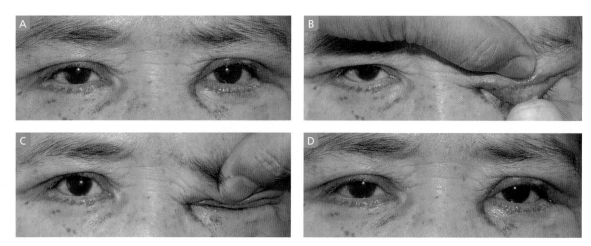

FIGURE 5-53 • Manual stretching of the overcorrected eyelid in the early postoperative period.
A. The left eyelid is higher than the right eyelid. **B.** While the patient tries to keep the eyes open, the eyelash is pulled downward. To minimize the tension across the incision line, the eyebrow is also brought down together. **C.** An easier method. While the patient is opening the eyelid, the eyebrow is pressed downward. **D.** The left eyelid is at a more even height.

eyelid height can increase fairly late for levator shortening. If the levator muscle is damaged, the levator function may slowly return over the period of a year, and improvements in lagophthalmos observed with tissue remodeling.

Mild overcorrection of ptosis can be mitigated by forced stretching via downward massaging of the upper eyelids within the first two weeks of operation. If the overcorrection is significant, the eyelid should be revised in the operating room in the early period. The massage is performed by downward pressure on the eyelid while the patient tries to keep the eyes open. Only the portion of eyelid superior to the crease is pressed to avoid pulling across the incision line. The eyelashes can also be pulled downward while the eyebrow is pulled downward as well, to relieve any stress on across the incision. The downward massaging works better for techniques that use smaller number of sutures, and does not work well for higher number of sutures (FIGURE 5-53).

The advantages of early revision over delayed revision are that the operation is technically less challenging, the degree of advancement is easier to figure out, no dissection is necessary, and that the delay in recovery time is minimal, which helps with maintaining an understanding rapport with the patient. A significant problem with delayed revision of retraction is the risk of corneal complication and of permanent lid lag. If overcorrection (i.e. lid retraction) is addressed several months after the initial operation, the levator complex will require a more complicated operation.

Early revision can be adjusted without much trouble. Because of these reasons, early revision is absolutely more advantageous.

Postoperative changes in visual acuity

Patients may complain about visual acuity change after blepharoplasty operations and, especially, ptosis correction.

The postoperative edema can lead to a temporary decrease in lacrimal function, and early ectropion may disrupt the Meibomian glands. The resulting xerophthalmia can not only cause discomfort but also decrease visual acuity. Chemosis is another cause of decrease in visual acuity.

Another frequent clinical problem is the development of astigmatism. This is caused by decreased contact pressure between the eyelid and the cornea. In most situations, the astigmatism resolves after 3 months. The proportion of patients who continue to experience astigmatism is reported to be low. Therefore, patients should be counseled on waiting for the visual acuity to improve, instead of obtaining new eyeglasses.

PTOSIS CORRECTION AND DOUBLE FOLD OPERATION

Double fold operation is different when it is combined with ptosis correction. The major issues are the height and depth of eyelid creases.

Design of double-fold crease in ptotic eyelid

An eyelid crease designed on a ptotic eyelid will be lower in the medial and central portion of the eyelid with the lateral portion relatively unaffected. This results in an eyelid crease that is narrower medially and wider laterally. Thus, eyelid crease needs to be designed with this in mind (FIGURE 5-54).

In non-ptotic eyelids, the height and shape of eyelid crease can be designed after the temporary eyelid crease made with a stylus. However, the same approach in a

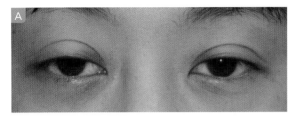
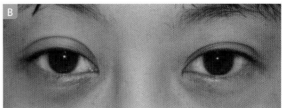

FIGURE 5-54 • **A.** Eyelid crease in a patient with ptosis. Overall, the eyelid crease is set high above the eyelid margin. The height is greatest in the middle and tapers laterally. **B.** The patient was instructed to open the eyelids with extra effort. The crease height has decreased significantly.

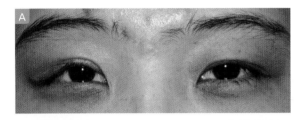

FIGURE 5-55 • **A.** Right ptosis. **B.** Left ptosis. Ectropion is present medially and centrally. The crease is non-existent laterally. **C.** Bilateral ptosis. Ectropion is present centrally, and the crease is faint laterally.

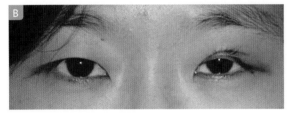
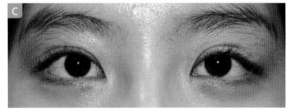

ptotic eyelid will result in lower fold. To simulate the effect of ptosis correction, the patient is instructed to open the eyelids as much as possible, while the eyebrow is fixed in a neutral position by an assistant during the design process.

It may be that severe ptosis prevents raising of the eyebrow even with maximal effort from the patient. In such cases, the design of the eyelid crease can begin in the lateral aspect, where the height of the eyelid crease does not change as much upon ptosis operation. The design is then extended medially, while respecting the curvature of crease.

Ptosis correction will usually result in a double fold that is wider laterally and thinner medially and centrally. The operator must be cautious of this.

Ectropion and faintness of crease is common for eyelid creases after ptosis correction. More specifically, deep eyelid crease (i.e. ectropion) is frequent in the central eyelid, and shallow eyelid crease (i.e. faintness) is frequent laterally (FIGURE 5-55).

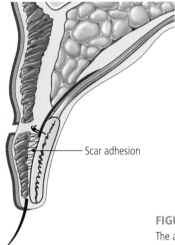

— Scar adhesion

FIGURE 5-56 • Mechanism by which ectropion occurs frequently after ptosis operation. The advanced levator aponeurosis can become connected to the skin indirectly through adhesion.

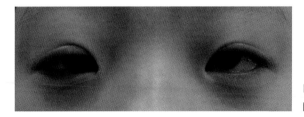

FIGURE 5-57 • The eyelid crease easily becomes undone after ptosis correction.

The reasons for ectropion are as follows:

1. The crease is fixated on levator aponeurosis that has been advance. As such, a neutrally placed suture actually represents a high fixation. This is the same reason for faint eyelid creases becoming deeply set with maximal eye opening.

2. During the advancement, the fixation suture may indirectly incorporate subcutaneous structures such as the orbicularis muscle. In such cases, the fixation of this pretarsal tissue can result in ectropion of the eyelid even before the eyelid crease sutures are placed. In effect, the advancement fixation sutures are connecting the posterior lamella and anterior lamella **(FIGURE 5-56)**.

Fixation of advanced levator to the tarsal plate will cause ectropion if there is any adhesion between the anterior lamella and posterior lamella because the force from levator muscle will transfer through the adhesion to the skin.

The disappearance of eyelid crease is also common **(FIGURE 5-57)**. This is because the ptotic eyelid is not dynamic but static. A natural eyelid crease tends to become faint with downgaze and is more noticeable in a neutral gaze. However, the crease

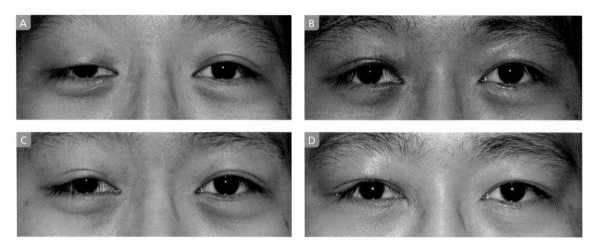

FIGURE 5-58 • A case of right-sided ptosis.
A. Preoperative photograph. **B.** After correction of right ptosis and creation of eyelid crease. **C.** Right eyelid is lower, and the eyelid crease has become shallow. **D.** After the second correction.

of a ptotic eyelid tends to remain statically bold at all times. Therefore, the crease height should be fixed carefully.

The solution to the problem of faint crease in the lateral eyelid

During ptosis correction, the levator aponeurosis is advanced only in central portion of the eyelid. Laterally, the aponeurosis advancement is usually skipped, and this is the area where the surgically created crease tends to become undone or end up high **(FIGURE 5-58)**. To prevent this, the lower skin flap should be fixated not only to the tarsal plate but also to a location higher on the aponeurosis, as if performing ptosis correction in the lateral portion of the eyelid **(FIGURE 5-59)**.

This lateral fixation for the crease can be thought of as creating a mechanism similar to aponeurosis advancement.

One commonly overlooked problem in ptosis correction and eyelid crease is that fixation of the lower flap can burden the lower portion of levator muscle, such that the eyelid margin is lowered. During the operation, fixation of the lower flap to the tarsal plate is associated with 0-to-1.5 mm of decrease in eyelid height. Because of this, creation of eyelid crease requires additional overcorrection in patients with ptosis.

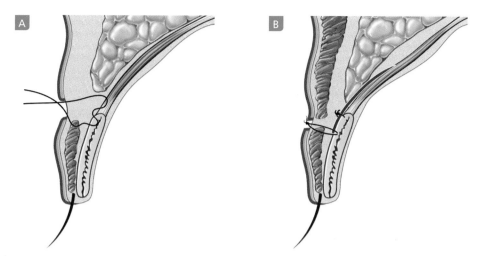

FIGURE 5-59 • **A.** Crease fixation in the lateral eyelid with ptosis. The 3-point fixation is performed between orbicularis muscle, tarsal plate, and levator aponeurosis. **B.** Crease fixation in the medial and central portion of the eyelid. The fixation is created between the lower portion of the tarsal plate and to the advanced levator aponeurosis.

In patients with pre-existing eyelid crease in only one side, it is more convenient to create the crease in the creaseless eyelid first before proceeding with the ptosis correction in both eyelids. If the ptosis correction is performed first, the creation of eyelid crease will lower that side. In ptosis correction, the operation is not complete until the crease has been fixated.

Taxation after ptosis correction

(The eyelid margin lowers after ptosis correction)

Because of the visual obstruction, patients with ptosis exert significant effort in raising the eyelid and eyebrow. The correction of ptosis improves much of the visual field deficit and removes the drive to open the eyelid and raise the eyebrow. This decrease in the drive results in a "laziness" of maintaining the eyelid height. In some cases, the ptotic eyelid appears to remain in the same position despite significant advancement in levator tissue. This can represent a failure of the operation or a change in the drive to keep the eyelids elevated. Such change in neuromuscular balance must be respected in ptosis surgery. This can also be observed during ptosis operation, where the advanced eyelid will loose some of the gained height. However, lowering of the eyelid height at a later stage in the operation is most likely due to edema. This inevitable decrease in the eyelid height during ptosis correction can be thought of as a tax on the profit of the labor.

In addition, ptosis correction has the effect of increasing eyelid thickness. Advancement of the levator muscle and aponeurosis will also advance the orbital fat, which adds to the overall thickness of the eyelid. After a ptosis operation, a hallow eyelid will become less hollow; a normal eyelid will be slightly full; and a full eyelid will become too full. In the latter case, the ptosis operation may necessitate orbital fat resection. In extreme cases, resection of orbital fat and other connective tissues is not enough to decrease the thickness of the eyelid. Another reason for eyelid thickness is the descent of soft tissue with lower eyebrows. In contrast, correction of retracted eyelid will elevate the orbital fat along with the aponeurosis, which will cause sunken eyelid. This also increases the risk of triple fold formation.

UPPER EYELID RETRACTION

Retraction refers to excessively high position of the upper eyelid. In a normal setting, about 1-to-2 mm of the upper corneal limbus is covered by the eyelid. Exposure of the topmost 1 mm of cornea or the exposure of sclera above it is considered as retraction. However, elderly patients sometimes wish to lower the eyelid even when the eyelid does not meet the criteria for retraction on physical exam.

Symptoms
- The appearance of surprise or anger
- Xerophthalmia
- Foreign body sensation
- Blurred vision
- Photophobia
- Ectropion or entropion

As with blepharoptosis, upper eyelid retraction can be divided into excessive function of the levator muscle (biologic) and physical advancement of the muscle (mechanical).

Biologic retraction includes hyperthyroidism or other primary retractions, and mechanical retraction includes complications of ptosis correction and trauma.

This categorization becomes a determining factor in the amount of extension required at the time of operation.

Techniques for eyelid retraction

- Müllerectomy
- Levator recession and levator lengthening
- Aponeurosis recession with or without Müllerectomy
- Spacer graft

Levator lengthening with pretarsal tissue

This technique is usually reserved for not-so-severe cases of retraction. Retraction from the complication of ptosis surgery is usually not so severe.

The local anesthesia, like in ptosis correction, begins with injection of 1% lidocaine with or without 1:100,000 epinephrine along the planned skin incision. Regional block is used for supraorbital nerve, supratrochlear nerve (1.0-1.5 ml), and lacrimal nerve (0.5-1.0 ml). Intraoperatively, additional doses of lidocaine without epinephrine may be used sparingly, while minimizing eyelid height changes.

Upon skin incision, the orbicularis muscle is divided, and the tarsal plate is exposed. The aponeurosis is separated from the septum. There are several methods of lengthening the levator muscle. Here, the author introduces a method of levator extension using the pretarsal soft tissue.

A small amount of lidocaine without epinephrine is injected into the pretarsal soft tissue. The pretaral soft tissue is dissected from 4-5 mm below the upper border of the tarsal plate. The dissection is carried superiorly. Anesthetic drops are applied to the eye, and normal saline is used to dissect the space between the Müller's muscle and conjunctiva. The Müller's muscle is separated from the tarsal plate. From the top, the muscle is dissected away from the conjunctiva. All of these maneuvers are designed such that the pretarsal tissue becomes an extension of the Müller's muscle. Prior to separating the Müller's muscle from conjunctiva, the eyelid height is evaluated for any anesthesia or edema-related changes. The dissection is carried medially and laterally, then superiorly. The eyelid height should be

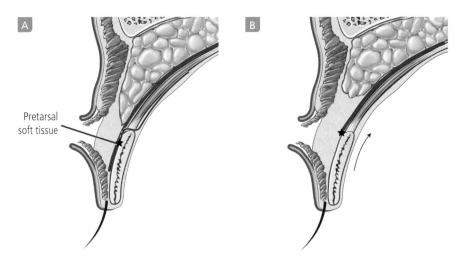

FIGURE 5-60 • Levator lengthening using the pretarsal tissue.
The pretarsal tissue is used as an extension, which allows the levator muscle to recede.

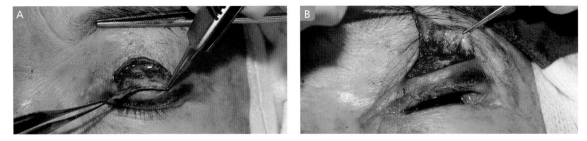

FIGURE 5-61 • This patient had a levator shortening operation, with levator muscle as the pretarsal tissue.

evaluated in incremental steps. The dissection is completed when the eyelid margin assumes a ptotic position.

Once the eyelid is in a ptotic position, the remainder of operation is relatively similar to ptosis correction. The pretarsal tissue is secured to the tarsal plate such that the eyelid height represents 0.5 mm of overcorrection, as it is with usual for ptosis surgery **(FIGURE 5-60)**. If the patient has a history of levator shortening, a remnant of the levator muscle may remain in the pretarsal area **(FIGURE 5-61)**. This structure is more robust than the usual pretarsal tissue, and in such cases, overcorrection of the ptosis may not be necessary **(FIGURE 5-62)**.

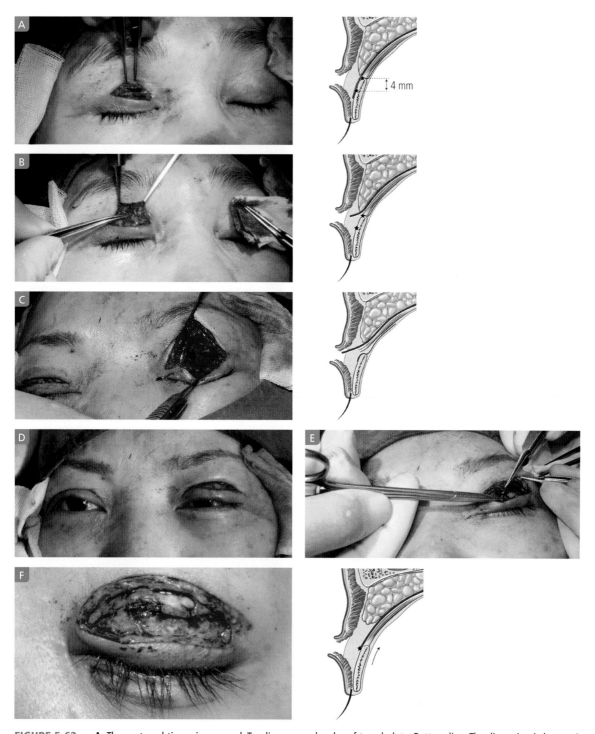

FIGURE 5-62 • **A.** The pretarsal tissue is exposed. Top line: upper border of tarsal plate. Bottom line: The dissection is begun 4 mm below the upper border. **B.** The pretarsal tissue is dissected from the tarsal plate. The lower forceps indicates the upper border of tarsal plate. **C.** The Müller's muscle is separated from the tarsal plate and is dissected from the conjunctiva. **D.** Dissection of Müller's muscle from conjunctiva has resulted in the ptosis of the eyelid. **E.** The lower end of dissected levator complex is secured to the tarsal plate. **F.** The end of pretarsal flap is receded 4 mm and secured onto the tarsal plate.

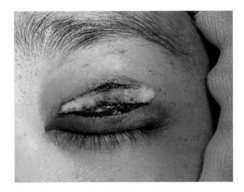

FIGURE 5-63 • Spacer graft made from Alloderm.

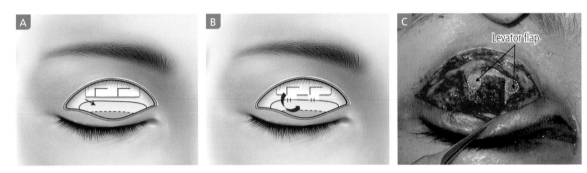

FIGURE 5-64 • Pretarsal tissue rotation flap. Illustration and intraoperative photograph.

Key points for levator lengthening

- At 4-5 mm below the upper border, the pretarsal tissue is separated away from the tarsal plate.
- Müller's muscle is separated from tarsal plate and conjunctiva.
- The dissection is carried out until the eyelid margin is ptotic.
- The pretarsal tissue is fixated to the tarsal plate. The eyelid is elevated for 1 mm of overcorrection.

The most commonly used corrective method for eyelid retraction is the spacer graft. Usually, correction of ptosis requires advancement that is 3-4 times the amount of ptosis. Correction of eyelid retraction requires spacer graft that is about 2 times the length of retraction. Source of spacer graft include autogenous tissues such as deep temporal fascia and hard palate mucosa and allografts like acellular dermal matrix **(FIGURE 5-63)**. Recommendations on graft widths have varied from 1 times to 2 times the amount of eyelid retraction. Spinelli used deep temporal fascia to extend the levator complex by 2 times the amount of retraction. McCord extended the levator by the equal degree of retraction. Fox used the sclera to extend the levator by 2 times the retraction. Berke corrected the retraction using levator tenotomy by 2 times the length. Lai and Piggot extended the levator by 2 times the length of retraction plus 2 mm.

Compared to autograft, allografts are more likely to become absorbed and cause tissue contraction, with subsequent recurrence in eyelid retraction.

Eyelids retractions as ptosis complication do not exceed more than 3 mm of retraction. As such, the pretarsal tissue is sufficient in extending the levator muscle in most cases. If the pretarsal tissue extension is not enough, however, the author employs levator rotation flap. It is important to make sure the levator flap is not too thin, as cheese-wiring of the flap can result in ptosis of the eyelid. To ensure the levator stays as thick as possible, the rotation are limited to just one or two flaps **(FIGURE 5-64)**.

Retractions from biologic causes such as hyperthyroidism are often more severe in the lateral aspect of eyelids. Recurrence of retraction is more common in the lateral eyelid, and ptosis is more frequent in the medial eyelid. Therefore, the dissection should begin from the lateral portion and be carried medially.

 WAIT A MINUTE!

AT TIMES, DISSECTION OF THE RETRACTED LEVATOR MUSCLE FROM CONJUNCTIVA DOES NOT LEAD TO A DECREASE IN EYELID HEIGHT. HOWEVER, THIS WILL CERTAINLY DEVELOP INTO PTOSIS IF LEFT ALONE. WHY IS THIS?

This observation can be explained by incomplete dissection. To exaggerate, just 2% of adhesion between levator and conjunctiva can withstand the weight of the eyelid. However, this will subsequently be followed by ptosis. From the ptotic position, the eyelid can be elevated to the proper height.

Advantages of eyelid retraction surgery using pretarsal tissue extension

- Technically less demanding
- Does not require a donor graft
- The spacer graft requires two rows of sutures whereas the pretarsal tissue

extension only requires a single row. This difference is helpful in reducing the variability in the eyelid height (more predictable).

- Revision is easier. The fixation point can easily be moved along the tarsal plate to adjust the eyelid height.

 WAIT A MINUTE!

CORRECTION OF PTOSIS REQUIRES ADVANCEMENT THAT IS 4 TIMES THE AMOUNT OF PTOSIS, BUT CORRECTION OF EYELID RETRACTION REQUIRES A RECESSION THAT IS ABOUT 2 TIMES THE LENGTH OF RETRACTION. WHY DOES THE AMOUNT OF MOVEMENT DIFFER BETWEEN PTOSIS AND RETRACTION?

The eyelid is a highly dynamic tissue that movements more than ten thousand times within a 24-hour period. This causes cheese-wiring of the tissue, which causes loosening of the fixation. This loosening of the fixation point causes descent of the eyelid after both types operations. Thus, ptosis correction must overcorrect for the fact that the eyelid will drop a big, whereas recession must undercorrect for the same reason. On one hand, a ptosis of 3 mm will be overcorrected by 4 mm, to account for the postoperative drop. On the other hand, a retraction of 3 mm will be undercorrected by 2 mm, to account for the 1 mm of postoperative drop in eyelid height.

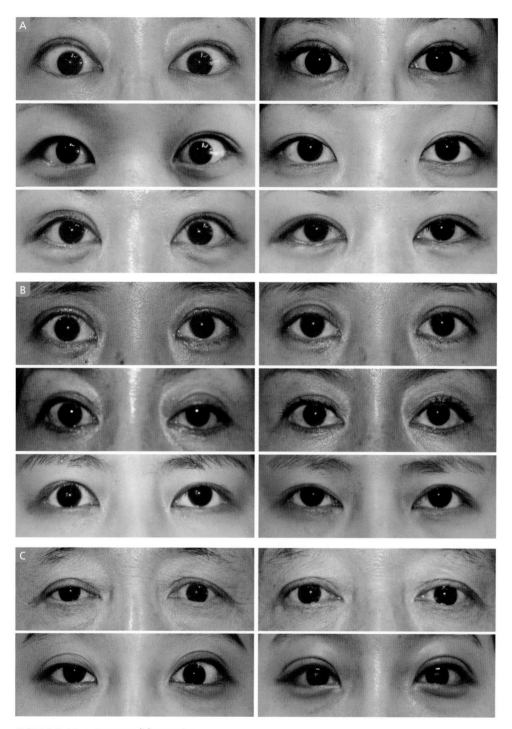

FIGURE 5-65 • Upper eyelid retraction.
A. Bilateral retraction. **B.** Unilateral retraction. **C.** Retraction and ptosis.

📑 REFERENCES

1. Fox SA : Surgery of ptosis. William & Wilkins. Baltimore. p.71, 1980.
2. Beard C : Ptosis(3rd ed.) St. Louis. C.V. Mosby Co. p.116, 1981.
3. Nahai F : The art of aesthetic surgery. St. Louis. Publishing, Inc. 2005.
4. Flower RS : The art of eyelid and orbital aesthetics : Multiracial surgical considerations. Clin Plast Surg 14:693, 1987.
5. Hoşal BM, Ayer NG, Zilelioğlu G, Elhan AH. Ultrasound biomicroscopy of the levator aponeurosis in congenital and aponeurotic blepharoptosis. Ophthal Plast Reconstr Surg 20:308, 2004.
6. Older JJ : Levator aponeurosis tuck : A treatment for ptosis. Ophthalmic Surg 9(4):102, 1978.
7. Older JJ : Levator aponeurosis surgery for the correction of acquired ptosis. Ophthamology 90:1056, 1983.
8. Doxanas MT : Simplified aponeurotic ptosis surgery. Ophthamic Surg 22(8):512, 1992.
9. Shao W, Byrne P, Harrison A, Nelson E, Hilger P : Persistent blurred vision after blepharoplasty and ptosis repair. Arch Facial Pastt Surg. 6:155-157, 2004.
10. Holck DE, Dutton JJ : Changes in astigmatism after ptosis surgery measured by corneal topography. Ophthal Plast Reconstr Surg 14(3):151-8, 1998.
11. Choi KS, Kim YS, Lee TS : A Clinical Study of Surgical Results on 466 Blepharoptosis. The Korean Ophthalmological Society 36:1093-104, 1995.
12. Chen WPD, Khan JA, McCord Jr. CD : Color Atlas of Cosmetic Oculofacial Surgery. Edinburgh, Butterworth Heinemann, Elsivier Science, 2004.
13. Lin KL, Uzcategui N, Chang EL : Effect of surgical correction of congenital ptosis on amblyopia. Ophthal Plast Recontr Surg 24(6):434-6.
14. Anderson RL, Baumgartner SA : Amblyopia in Ptois. Arch Ophthalmol 98:1068-9, 1980.
15. Holmstrom H, Santanelli F : Suspension of the eyelid to the check ligament of the superior fornix for congenital blepharoptosis. Scand J Plas Recontr Surg Hand Surg 36:149-56, 2002.
16. Song R, Song Y : Treatment of blepharoptosis ; Direct transplantation of frontalis muscle to upper eyelid. Clin Plast Surg 9:45, 1982.
17. Park DM, Song JW, Han KH, Kang JS : Anthropometry on Normal Korean Eyelids. Archives of Plastic Surgery 17:822-41, 1990.
18. Hwang K, Huan F, Kim Dj, Hwang S H. Size of the superior palpebral involuntary muscle (Müller muscle), J craniofacial surg 21(5):1626-9, 2010.
19. Soserburg GL : Kinesiology; Application to pathological motion. Baltimore: William & Wilkins, 1986.
20. Cho I C, Kang J H, Kim K K. Correcting upper eyelid retraction by means of pretarsal levator lengthening for complications following ptosis surgery, Plast Reconst Surg 130(1):73-81.
21. Spinelli HM : Atlas of Aesthetic Eyelid Periocular Surgery. Elserier health Sciences, 2004.
22. Anderson RL, Beard C : The levator aponeurosis attachments and their clinical significance. Arch Ophthalmol. 95:1437-41, 1977.
23. Burman S, Betharia SM, Bajaj MS, et al. : AlOC Proceedings. Orbit Oculoplasty 1:441, 2002.
24. Harris WA, Dortzbach RK : Levator tuck : a simplified belpharoptosis procedure. Ann Opthalmol 7:873-8, 1975.
25. Jones LT, Quickert MH, Wobig JL : The cure of ptosis by aponeurotic repair. Arch Ophthalmol 93:629-34, 1975.
26. Liu D : Ptosis repair by single suture aponeurosis tuck. Surgical technique and long term results. Ophthalmology 100:251-9, 1993.
27. H. kakizaki, Y iakahashi : Muller's Muscle tendon : Microscopic Anatomy in Asians. Ophthal Plast Reconstr Surg. Vol.27. No2. 122-124.
28. Berke RN : Histology of levotor muscle in conqenital and acfuired ptosis. Arch Ophthalmol 53:413-28, 1955.
29. Kuwabara T : structure of muscle of upper eyelid. Arch Ophthalmol 93:1189-97, 1975.
30. Wolfley. De : Preventing conjunctival prolapse and tarsal evesion following large excisions of levator muscle and aponeurosis after correction of corgenital ptosis. Ophthalmic surg 18:491-4, 1987.
31. Francis CS : Histological changes in congenital and acquired blepharoptosis. Eye(2):179-84, 1988.
32. Hwang K, Shin YH, Kim DJ : Conjoint Fascial Sheath of the Levator and Superior Rectus attached to the conjunctival fornix. The J of Craniofacial Surgery 19(1):241-5, 2008.

06

LOWER BLEPHAROPLASTY WITH MIDFACE LIFT

- The aging process and various solutions
- Anatomy of the lower eyelid
- Operation procedure
- Periorbital fat
- Lower lid retraction
- Postoperative management
- Complications of lateral canthoplasty
- Lower eyelid entropion

THE AGING PROCESS AND VARIOUS SOLUTIONS

The aging process of the lower eyelid can be summarized by gravitational descent and volume loss of the connective tissue. However, age-related changes can appear in a wide varied of ways, and each change requires appropriate choice of operative technique.

The common problems of aging process can be associated to the operations performed to correct each problem. Various combinations of age-related changes can be addressed by a number of operative techniques. Below are comprehensive lists of lower blepharoplasty techniques and respective indications.

Various changes in aging periorbital structures

- Palpebral bags
- Nasojugal fold, palpebromalar fold
- Dark circle, dark pigmentation around eyes
- Infraorbital hollowness
- Skin wrinkles and skin redundancy
- Malar mound, malar crescent
- Pretarsal flatness
- Orbicularis oculi muscle hypertrophy
- Lid laxity – lid horizontal laxity and canthal tendon laxity
- Scleral show, ectropion
- Secondary blepharoplasty case
- Malar hypoplasia
- Exophthalmos or enophthalmos
- Crow's feet
- Mid-cheek groove, descent of the mid-cheek junction
- Nasolabial fold

Operative solutions

The various changes to lower eyelid are addressed by a wide spectrum of operative techniques. Among the various techniques listed below, a single procedure may be sufficient for an age-related change, but it's more common that a combination of procedures is indicated during a single operation. Procedures should be selected based on appropriate indications for each individual patient.

- Transconjunctival fat removal, transconjunctival fat reposition
- Skin resurfacing
- Filler injection, fat injection
- Skin, muscle excision
- Orbicularis oculi muscle suspension
- Canthal anchoring: canthoplasty, canthopexy
- Tarsal segmental excision
- Sub-orbicularis oculi fat elevation, levator labii superioris elevation
- Mid-cheek lifting
- Secondary blepharoplasty
- Retractor release
- Spacer graft

Aging process is accepted as a natural phenomenon. However, the undeniable situation is that this natural phenomenon of aging has a detrimental effect in leading a socially active life. On the sole basis of appearing older, talented people with valuable life experience are shunned and neglected by the greater society, which they have helped to build. This is not just a great tragedy for each aging person but also represents a tremendous waste of valuable human capital for our society. Thus, the pursuit of rejuvenation for the aging person becomes an issue of individual survival - the will to participate and live a relevant life in the greater society.

Therefore, the surgeon must keep in mind how an elderly person receiving upper and lower blepharoplasty must function within the society. In this context, the goal of rejuvenation is not simply to appear younger and beautiful but should be to rehabilitate the person to maintain or restore the social function.

Lower blepharoplasty can achieve satisfactory outcomes with excision of redundant skin and pseudoherniating fat. To maximize the benefit of operation and to minimize the risk of complications, however, a more individualized strategy may require a wide variety of operations. The increase in mean lifespan has increased the mean age of patients who wish to undergo aesthetic operation. And the increase in the number of male patients, who typically have worse outcomes than do female patients, also contributes to the likelihood of complications occurring after blepharoplasty. In addition, the increasing expectation regarding the advancement in medicine has lead to a societal pressure on the physicians who must meet the increased demand for positive outcomes, which tends to increase rates of complication following lower blepharoplasty.

In this chapter, the author wishes to introduce the spectrum of operations without delineating between primary and secondary operations. At times, operations designed for revisional surgery are indicated for primary operations.

In certain cases, midface lift is performed at the time of lower blepharoplasty. The author most commonly performs mini-midface lift in most elderly patients with broad midface lift reserve for occasional cases.

Simultaneous midface correction can 1) be more effective than blepharoplasty alone, 2) alleviate infraorbital hollowness by sub-orbicularis oculi fat (SOOF), 3) be effective in correcting the nasolabial fold, and 4) prevent and even treat complications of lower blepharoplasty such as lower eyelid retraction. However, one must also bear in mind that midface lift is also a causative factor for lower eyelid retraction.

In lower blepharoplasty, the surgeon must understand of the anatomy and be familiar with the structural characteristics above all else.

ANATOMY OF THE LOWER EYELID (FIGURE 6-1)

In non-pathologic state, the lower eyelid margin just touches or covers up to 1 mm of the lower limbus of cornea. Additionally, the line from medial canthus to the lateral canthus has an upward slope. This slope is called the canthal tilt, and the degree of this slope varies according to age, sex, and race. Compared to Caucasian populations, this line is steeper in East Asian populations. In this population, the lateral canthus is approximately 3-to-5 mm higher than the medial canthus, which translates to a 5-10 degree of canthal tilt (FIGURE 6-2).

The lower eyelid can be divided into three layers.

The anterior lamella contains skin and orbicularis oculi muscle.

The middle lamella contains the septum.

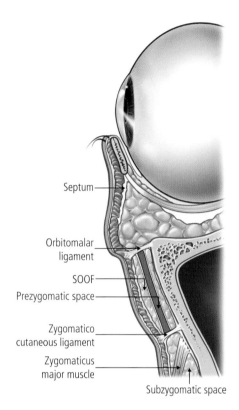

Septum

Orbitomalar ligament

SOOF

Prezygomatic space

Zygomatico cutaneous ligament

Zygomaticus major muscle

Subzygomatic space

FIGURE 6-1 • Anatomy of the lower eyelid.

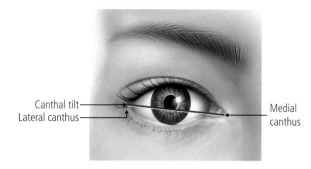

Canthal tilt
Lateral canthus

Medial canthus

FIGURE 6-2 • The lower eyelid and canthal tilt.

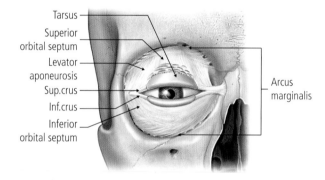

Tarsus
Superior orbital septum
Levator aponeurosis
Sup.crus
Inf.crus
Inferior orbital septum

Arcus marginalis

FIGURE 6-3 • Lower eyelid structures.
Superior orbital septum, Inferior orbital septum, tarsal plate, inferior crus, superior crus, medial and lateral canthal tendons, arcus marginalis.

The posterior lamella contains, with the tarsoligamentous sling as the center, the lower lid retractor (capsulopalpebral fascia and inferior tarsal muscle) and the conjunctiva. At times, the eyelid is considered in two layers, with the septum being considered as a part of the posterior lamella. The two retractors pull down on the lower eyelid to improve the visual field during downgaze.

In East Asian patients, the tarsal plates are 8-9 mm tall in the upper eyelid and 3-4 mm in the lower eyelid. The plates are connected to the lateral canthus by superior and inferior crus **(FIGURE 6-3)**.

The lateral canthus is composed of lateral canthal tendon and lateral retinaculum. The lateral canthal tendon is a complex connective tissue framework with a length of 4-7 mm (Hwang and 2 mm in thickness). Depending on the report, the lateral retinaculum is considered as the lateral canthus itself, with the tendon as a portion of the retinaculum **(FIGURE 6-4)**.

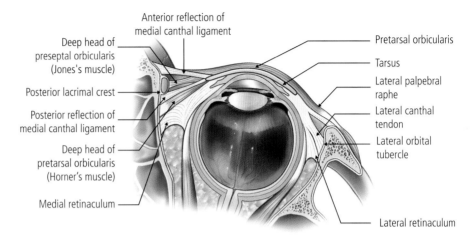

FIGURE 6-4 • Anatomy of lateral canthus.

The structure of lateral retinaculum

- Lateral canthal tendon
- Lateral horn of levator aponeurosis
- Whitnall's ligament
- Inferior suspensory ligament (Lockwood ligament)
- Check ligament of lateral rectus muscle

OPERATION PROCEDURE

Preoperative evaluation of the lower lid laxity (FIGURE 6-5)

- Snap back test
- Distraction test
- Pinch test

The snap back test evaluates the velocity at which the lower eyelid returns to the globe after having been depressed with the examiner's hand. Lid laxity is suspected if the eyelid does not instantaneously return to its original position.

The distraction test is performed by pulling on the lower eyelid and observing the distance between the globe and the eyelid. The normal distance is 3-to-5 mm,

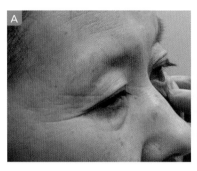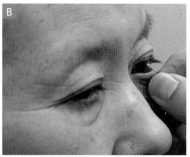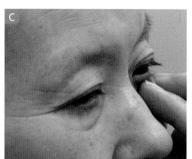

FIGURE 6-5 • Demonstration of lower lid laxity evaluations.
A. Snap back test. **B.** Distraction test. **C.** Pinch test.

whereas lid laxity is suspect for 6-to-7 mm.

The pinch test is performed by pinching the middle portion of the eyelid. Centralization of the lateral portion of the eyelid is suggestive of canthal weakening (dehiscence, disinsertion, or lengthening).

Operative steps

- Skin incision
- Subcutaneous and submuscular dissection
- Mobilization of orbital fat
- Dissection of midface
- Elevation of sub-orbicularis oculi fat
- Lateral canthal anchoring
- Suspension of orbicularis oculi muscle
- Formation of pretarsal fullness
- Skin closure

Skin incision and dissection of subcutaneous and submuscular planes

The lower eyelid skin is incised 2-3 mm inferior to the eyelashes. Laterally, the incision is extended inferolaterally into one of the wrinkles in the crow's feet. The extension should assume not an acute but an obtuse angle, in order to prevent the formation of webbing in the lateral eyelid **(FIGURE 6-64)**. Medially, extension of incision medial to the lacrimal punctum can prevent the formation of dog ear when significant amount of skin is excised. Here, the skin excision must not incorporate excision of the orbicularis muscle.

The advantage of 2-3 mm offset incision

Some surgeons have stated that the transcutaneous incision should be as close to the eyelashes as possible. However, an incision that is offset from the eyelashes is preferable for the following reasons.

1. The skin is fairly thin from the eyelid margin to within 1-2 mm of the orbital rim and becomes significantly thicker below the rim. If the incision is made in the thin portion of eyelid skin, the skin closure will become uneven because of the mismatch to the skin from below, in terms of color, texture, and thickness. However, such incisions does not lead to mismatched skin closure in those occasional patients with relatively thick eyelid skin.

2. In some patients, a severe depression can be observed 2 mm below the eyelashes, which must be avoided at the time of incision.

3. Incisions just close to the eyelid margin can result in ectropion even with the slightest amount of skin tension.

Once the skin is incised, the dissection is carried in the subcutaneous plane. The subcutaneous dissection is carried widely in the lateral eyelid but is maintained narrowly in the medial portion. The subcutaneous dissection is maintained superficial to the pretarsal oculi muscle. Inferior to the tarsal plate, the dissection is carried deep to the orbicularis muscle. In patients with pretarsal hollowness, the incision through the orbicularis muscle should be made lower as to allow incorporation of more muscle in the superior flap. The medial 1-cm of orbicularis muscle should not be divided to protect the buccal branch of the facial nerve, which innervates procerus muscle and the medial pretarsal orbicularis muscle.

Upon incision of the orbicularis muscle, the dissection is carried in the submuscular plane. The pretarsal oculi muscle maintains the tone and position of the lower eyelid and stabilizes the tarsal plate. The medial portion of this muscle is especially important because it allows for blinking of the eyelids as well as lacrimal secretion. Thus, the pretarsal oculi muscle must be preserved during the dissection. In most cases, the orbicularis muscle is divided about 4-5 mm inferior to the lower border of the tarsal plate, and the dissection is carried in the submuscular plane **(FIGURE 6-6)**.

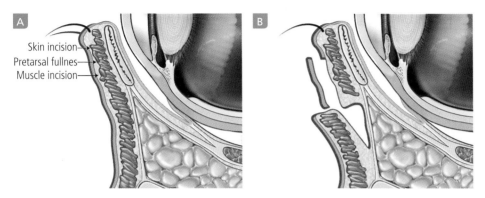

Skin incision
Pretarsal fullnes
Muscle incision

FIGURE 6-6 • Skin incision, orbicularis oculi muscle incision, and sub-muscular dissection. Anterior to the tarsal plate, the dissection is carried in the subcutaneous plane. Inferior to the tarsal plate, the dissection is carried in the sub-muscular plane.

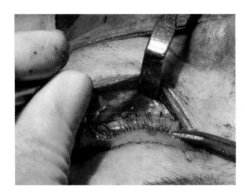

FIGURE 6-7 • The dissection between oculi muscle and orbital septum has been carried down to the orbital rim.

If the orbicularis muscle is incised too high, the inferior tarsal arcade could become injured, and the pretarsal area might become hollow. The submuscular dissection is extended inferiorly to the orbital rim, and the muscle flap is elevated **(FIGURE 6-7)**. The plane between orbicularis muscle and the orbital septum is dissected using cotton or blunt tip of an instrument to minimize the risk of injury to the orbital septum, to prevent orbital fat herniation and septal scarring.

Arcus marginalis release

At the orbital rim, the orbital septum joins the periosteum to form the arcus marginalis, which is released through the dissected space. The dissection is then carried in either the supra-periosteal or sub-periosteal plane. Medially, the orbicularis muscle is tightly adhered to the periosteum by the tear-through ligament and this

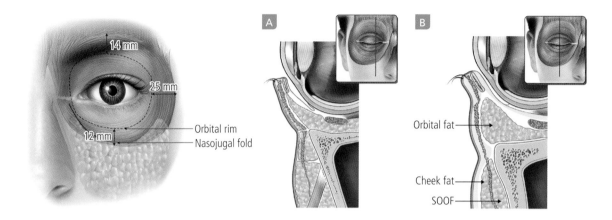

FIGURE 6-8 • Nasojugal fold.
A. The medial border is defined by the attachment between the orbicularis muscle and the periosteum. **B.** Laterally, the orbicularis retaining ligament is connected to the periosteum, and the orbicularis oculi muscle is attached to the periosteum at a point lower than the orbital septum, which forms nasojugal fold. Also, the nasojugal fold coincides as the upper border of cheek fat and as the transition point between the preseptal and preorbital portions of the orbicularis muscle. Therefore, the transposition of orbital fat into the space created after dissection of the fold serves to augment the volume into the depressed area and to prevent re-adhesion.

adhesion should be divided. Laterally to this, the orbicularis muscle is connected indirectly to the orbital rim via the orbitomalar ligament. Orbitomalar ligament originates from the periosteum just inferior to the orbital rim and pierces through the orbicularis muscle to attach to the skin. Depending on the location, the ligament varies in length. It is longest at the midpupillary line and becomes shorter laterally. At the lateral canthus, it becomes the lateral orbital thickening.

Nasojugal fold has the following characteristics.

- Medially, the fold is defined by the attachment between the orbicularis muscle and the periosteum **(FIGURE 6-8)**.
- Centrally, the fold is defined by the attachment between orbitomalar ligament and the skin **(FIGURE 6-8)**.
- The fold demarcates the superior border of the cheek fat **(FIGURE 6-8)**.
- The fold also demarcates the transition between the thin, pretarsal portion of the orbicularis muscle to the thicker, preorbital portion.

Therefore, the transposition of orbital fat into the space created after dissection of the fold serves to augment the volume into the depressed area and to prevent re-adhesion.

Correction of pretarsal depression or flatness
Restoration of pretarsal fullness

The author's technique
The author's method of creating pretarsal fullness is accomplished by bunching of pretarsal orbicularis muscle and of pretarsal orbicularis muscle. In this technique, the pretarsal orbicularis lower edge of the muscle is fixated at a higher position to cause bunching of the muscle mass. Then, the preorbital muscle is then brought up to overlap the bunched pretarsal muscle mass. The location of pretarsal fullness is crucial. The width of pretarsal fullness is also important, as too wide of a pretarsal fullness can appear less than sophisticated. To place the pretarsal fullness high in the lower eyelid, the pretarsal orbicularis muscle should be bunched thick. The orbicularis muscle is divided 2-to-3 mm below the pretarsal fullness, and the submuscular dissection will allow the pretarsal muscle flap to be bunched (FIGURE 6-9).

In younger persons, the pretarsal fullness is present at all times and becomes thicker and more noticeable with certain facial expressions. With aging, the pretarsal orbicularis muscle looses tone, and the muscle and connective tissue can undergo atrophy and/or descent. These changes lead to flatness or hollowness of the area, which is one of the hallmarks of facial aging (FIGURE 6-10). Therefore, surgical recovery of the pretarsal fullness is important for youthful appearance.

Operative details
- An adequate amount of pretarsal orbicularis muscle should be available for tissue bulking.
- The preseptal orbicularis muscle is brought up and suspended in front of the preseptal orbicularis muscle. The addition of midface lift is very effective at this point.
- The skin is closed with interrupted 6-0 nylon sutures. Each suture is driven through the skin, preseptal orbicularis muscle, inferior edge of pretarsal muscle, and again through the skin. This causes the pretarsal muscle to bunch upward (FIGURE 6-9C).

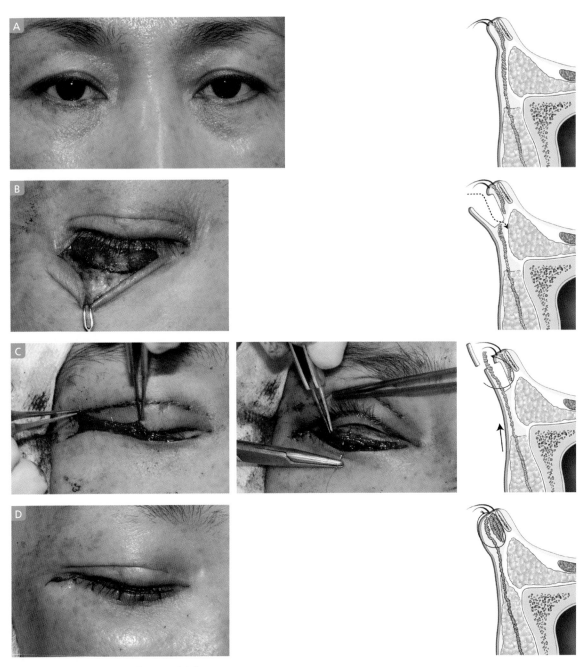

FIGURE 6-9 • Formation of pretarsal fullness.
A. Preoperative photograph. **B.** Upon skin incision, the subcutaneous dissection is carried inferiorly until 4-5 mm below the tarsal plate. At this point, the dissection is continued in the submuscular plane. To create bunching of tissue, the orbicularis muscle is divided in the preseptal portion. **C.** Left: After skin excision, the preseptal orbicularis muscle can be observed. Right: The suture is passed from beneath the pretarsal orbicularis muscle, which causes the bunch of tissue. The preseptal orbicularis muscle is laid on top of the bunched pretarsal tissue. **D.** Pretarsal fullness after the fixation.

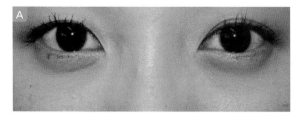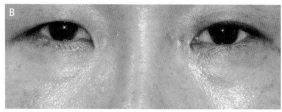

FIGURE 6-10 • Comparison of pretarsal fullness between younger and older persons.

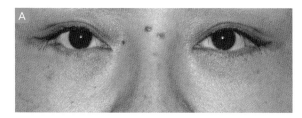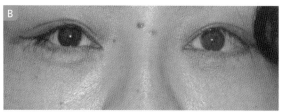

FIGURE 6-11 • Photograph of before and after Alloderm implantation for pretarsal fullness.

- The skin is closed without excessive tension.
- The suspension of the orbicularis oculi muscle tightens the muscle.

An important factor in successful creation of pretarsal fullness is the tensionless closure of the skin. If the skin closure is too tight, the consolidation of orbicularis muscle mass is not effective. The wrinkles in the skin should not be addressed by excision of the skin but is corrected by suspension of orbicularis muscle. Therefore, skin excision should be conservative with adequate amount of lower lid skin reserved for tensionless closure.

This method is effective in those who have lost the pretarsal fullness of youth. However, the method is not as effective in patients who never had pretarsal fullness in youth or has lost the fullness from excision of the pretarsal orbicularis muscle in a previous operation. In such patients, autogenous or allogeneic dermal graft is recommend **(FIGURE 6-11)**.

Cheek-midface lift

This technique elevates the midface and suspends it to the central or lateral portion of the orbital wall and has various effects.

- The operation corrects the descent of midface.
- Medially, the orbicularis oculi muscle and sub-orbicularis oculi fat is lifted, which corrects the infraorbital hollowness.
- Deep to the orbicularis muscle is the sub-orbicularis oculi fat. Superficial to the muscle is the malar fat and cheek fat. The mobilization of these orbicularis oculi muscle is effective at improving the malar crescent and nasolabial fold. Therefore the orbicularis oculi muscle is considered the handle of midface lifting.
- Restoration of tension to the preseptal oculi muscle is helpful in controlling the pseudoherniation of the orbital fat.
- In patients with lower lid retraction, the skin shortage is supplemented by oculi muscle upward suspension.
- The lifted midface tissue buttresses the lateral canthus in the desired postoperative position, as a canthal anchoring support.

Compared to conventional face lift, the midface lift via lower blepharoplasty has a more vertical vector and is therefore more effective. Also, the operation is more secure because the orbicularis oculi muscle can be fixated to the robust connective tissue (i.e. orbital wall periosteum or the deep temporal fascia).

Operative details

Through the steps detailed above, the dissection is carried between the orbicularis muscle and the orbital septum to the orbital rim, where the arcus marginalis is released. Medially, the orbicularis muscle is dissected free from the periosteum. Centrally and laterally, the muscle must be freed from the orbicularis retaining ligament, which serves as an indirect connection to the periosteum. Once the muscle is freed, the space between sub-orbicularis oculi fat and the periosteum can easily be dissected. The lateral attachment of the orbicularis retaining ligament is referred to as the lateral orbital thickening. Division of the lateral orbital thickening allows access to the zygomatico-facial ligament (zygomatic cutaneous ligament) next to the zygomatico-facial nerve. Dissection of this ligament allows relative mobilization of the midface. At this point, the dissection can be carried in the subperiosteal or

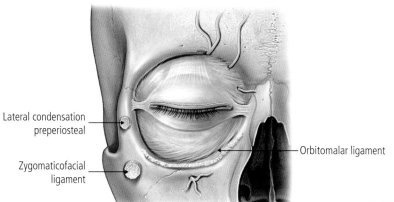

Lateral condensation preperiosteal

Zygomaticofacial ligament

Orbitomalar ligament

FIGURE 6-12 • Zygomaticofacial ligament.

supraperiosteal plane.

Supraperiosteal dissection

At the inferior margin, the dissection is carried between the periosteum and the sub-orbicularis oculi fat. Taking care not to injure the infraorbital nerve, the dissection is carried superficial to the levator labii superioris muscle medially and between the preperiosteal fat and the sub-orbicularis oculi fat. Below the orbital rim, the major and minor zygomatic muscle can be seen inserting into the bone. Near this point, the zygomatico-cutaneous ligament connects between zygomatic bone and the skin. Division of this ligament allows continued dissection down to the beginning of the alveolar bone **(FIGURE 6-12)**.

During midface lift, the mobilization of midfacial skin is more effective when the skin flap is thin. If the flap is thick, the deeper tissue may mobilize. However, the superficial layers (i.e. skin and orbicularis muscle) will be resistant to upward advancement. Because of this, the author tends to dissect the prezygomatic space to free the anterior layers and reserve the subperiosteal dissection in the presence of scar tissue **(FIGURES 6-13 and 6-14)**. According to Mendelson et al., prezygomatic space has orbicularis retaining ligament as the superior border, zygomaticocutaneous ligament as the inferior border, levator labii superioris as the medial border, zygomatic bone as the lateral border, the sub-orbicularis oculi fat as the anterior border, and the preperiosteal fat as the posterior wall. With respect to the prezygomatic space, the skin and sub-orbicularis oculi fat tends to droop anteriorly, whereas the preperiosteal fat and periosteum adheres strongly to the bone and does not descend with

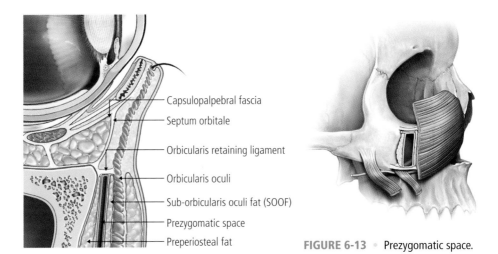

- Capsulopalpebral fascia
- Septum orbitale
- Orbicularis retaining ligament
- Orbicularis oculi
- Sub-orbicularis oculi fat (SOOF)
- Prezygomatic space
- Preperiosteal fat

FIGURE 6-13 • Prezygomatic space.

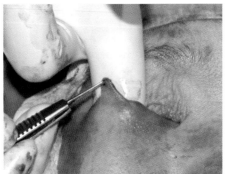

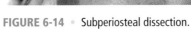

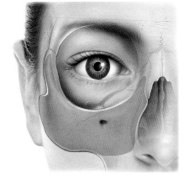

FIGURE 6-14 • Subperiosteal dissection.

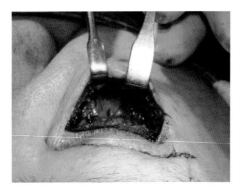

FIGURE 6-15 • Supraperiosteal dissection.
The dissection opens the space between preperiosteal fat and sub-orbicularis oculi fat. The preperiosteal fat can be observed in the floor of operative field.

aging. For this reason, the posterior lamella of the midface does not require significant lifting, and a thinner flap allows more upward mobilization of the anterior layers. Because of this, the author prefers the dissection in the preperiosteal plane (**FIGURE 6-15**). Thin flaps are especially useful in the patients with scleral show from lack of adequate skin. The advantage of prezygomatic space dissection is relatively atraumatic and because the flap is thinner, elevation of midface is more effective (**FIGURE 6-13**).

The actual dissection does not require cutting of connective tissue. Rather, the free space should be created by the spreading motion of blunt-tipped scissors. The elevator can be used to stretch the tissue, which will demonstrate a significant degree of elasticity. The method is relatively simple and fast, maintains hemostasis, and has a relatively lower risk of injury to the facial nerve branches. The edema is mild, and recovery is quick.

Subperiosteal dissection

A horizontal incision is made through the periosteum at 5 mm below the inferior orbital rim, leaving a cuff of periosteum on the orbital rim to provide a space to secure the suspension sutures. The subperiosteal space is entered through the incision. Medially, the dissection is carried beneath the levator labii superioris to the nasomaillary suture line. Laterally, the dissection is carried through the zygomatico-facial ligament to the zygomatico-maxillary suture line and inferior to malar retaining ligament, while preserving the lateral orbital thickening and the zygomatico-facial nerve. East Asian patients tend to find lateral prominence of the zygoma to be unattracted, and as such, dissections are not carried far out past the lateral orbital rim. The dissection is carried down towards the inferior margin of

TABLE 6-1 • Subperiosteal dissection VS Supraperiosteal dissection.

Subperiosteal dissection	Supraperiosteal dissection
Less bleeding. Arterial insufficiency to the midfacial tissue is not frequent.	More bleeding. Arterial insufficiency to the midfacial tissue can occur.
Atraumatic. Risk of injury to facial nerve is low.	Relative increase in tissue injury. Risk of injury to facial nerve is moderate.
Low elasticity	High elasticity
Dissection is easy but must be wide.	Dissection does not need to be wide.
Appropriate for patients with prior history of supraperiosteal dissection.	Effective in conservative surgery

the malar bone. The periosteal elevator is advanced until the instrument tip can be palpated via the index finger inserted in the buccal sulcus. The dissection is complete when the periosteum can be mobilized independently of the malar and alveolar bones. Near the alveolar bone, the periosteum is thin or dehisced, and the periosteum stretches easily without any relaxing incisions. If the dissection is not wide, relaxing incisions are needed to stretch the periosteum. The author does not recommend dividing the zygomatico-facial nerve to ease the dissection. However, division of the nerve leads to a minor and/or temporary sensory deficit.

Compared to the supraperiosteal space, the subperiosteal space is relatively avascular and can be dissected with relative ease. However, the tissue is relatively inelastic and requires wide dissection and/or relaxing incisions for adequate stretching. Generally, a midface flap is considered approximately 1.5 times more elastic without the periosteum. (Hamra) Supraperiosteal dissection has a higher potential for tissue trauma but yields a flap that is much more elastic without the periosteum and without the need for a wide dissection. Supraperiosteal dissection also yields a thinner flap, which is advantageous for augmenting the lack of lower eyelid skin. When elevating the sub-orbicularis oculi fat and the orbicularis muscle, thicker flaps tend to be restrictive in how much of the tissue can be lifted. The difference between subperiosteal and supraperiosteal dissections can be likened to the difference in footwear needed for light walking (supraperiosteal) versus heavy hiking (subperiosteal) for difficult terrain (secondary operation with tissue scar). In secondary cases with significant scarring, subperiosteal dissection is relatively atraumatic and avascular.

Midface lift operations have a toll fee

After midface lift, there is a high likelihood of lagophthalmos or scleral show. However, midface lift is also used to augment the lower eyelid skin to correct scleral show. Thus, midface lift is paradoxical in that it can both be a cause of and a correction for the insufficiency in lower eyelid skin. This is caused by postoperative scar contracture from wide dissection and especially from traumatic dissection and hematoma. Correction of skin shortage with midface lift should take into account the extra advancement required for postoperative scar contracture. Thus, entering the midface has a standard toll (scar contracture), and the operator must strive to obtain a greater value out of that toll.

Fat transposition

The pseudoherniated orbital fat is either excised or repositioned (septal reset) depending on the presence or absence of the nasojugal fold. Fat transposition is also helpful in correcting tear trough.

The tear trough exists as the border between preseptal and preorbital portion of the orbicularis oculi muscle, which is attached to the periosteum. It also coincides with the boundaries of the cheek fat (FIGURE 6-8), and fat transposition serves not only to augment the hollow area below the eyelids but also prevents re-adhesion of between the muscle and the periosteum. The fat is transposed beneath the lifted orbicularis muscle medially and beneath the sub-orbicularis oculi fat centrally. The central fat pad is transposed medially, after releasing any attachments to the orbital septum. A portion of the fat pad can be excised, or it can be repositioned if the palpebro-malar fold is distinct. The lateral fat should be examined after canthal anchoring, as it can bulge after the procedure. Also, the lower eyelid must be examined for height change due to fat transposition. If the eyelid margin is lower, it must be freed from any restraining elements such as the orbital septum, as transposition of orbital fat can result in eyelid retraction.

The orbital septum can be transposed with the fat for septal tightening, or the septum can be incised and the orbital fat can be transposed alone. The septum is loose in most cases, and the author prefers the simultaneous mobilization of the septum and fat. When the septum is being mobilized, the lower eyelid must be evaluated for retraction from the septum.

To evaluate which orbital fat must be transposed, the nasojugal fold and palpebral malar fold are marked. The infraorbital hollowness inferior to these lines is augmented by transposition of the fat to 5 mm below the fold. Centrally, nasojugal fold is about 1 cm below the inferior orbital rim (FIGURE 6-16). The nasojugal fold is 1) the border of the cheek fat of the anterior lamella and 2) the transition between the thin preseptal oculi muscle and the thicker preorbital oculi muscle. This is the main cause behind the transition from thin anterior lamella to thick anterior lamella. (Haddock) Intraoperatively, palpation of the dissected anterior lamella reveals this transition. In patients with defined nasojugal fold or with acute thickness transition, the orbital fat is repositioned just inferior to the transition in the thickness (FIGURE 6-17). This information regarding the appropriate location for fat transposition is also useful for fat injection.

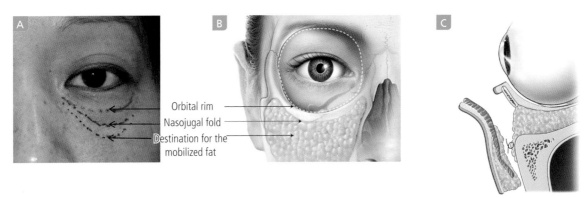

FIGURE 6-16 • Fat transposition.
A. Nasojugal fold and palpebromalar fold coincides with the upper border of cheek fat. Medially, the orbicularis muscle adheres directly to the orbital rim. **B.** The destination of transposed fat is 4-to-5 mm below the nasojugal fold. **C.** The transposed fat and lifted sub-orbicularis oculi fat.

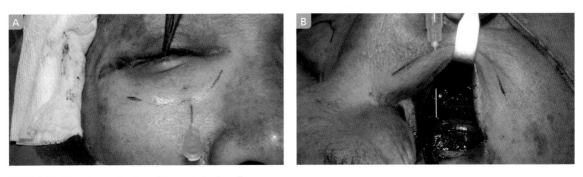

FIGURE 6-17 • Repositioning of the anterior lamella.
A. A needle is inserted through the nasojugal fold. **B.** The needle tip serves as a reference marker for fat repositioning.

A small portion of excessive fat herniation can be excised, but it is rare to excise the remaining fat after transposition. Excessive resection of fat can 1) cause depression in the lower eyelid, 2) contribute to enophthalmia and downward displacement of the globe, which can subsequently cause 3) hollowness of the upper eyelid from increased space between the orbital ceiling and 4) form adhesion between the septum and the capsulopalpebral fascia **(FIGURE 6-18B)**. The fat between the septum and the capsulopalpebral fascia acts as a ball bearing, and too large of an excision can cause direct contact and adhesion between the orbital septum and the capsulo-palpebral fascia. Postoperative inflammatory reaction to the septum does not cause much problem if the orbital fat is present. The absence of this fat, however, can

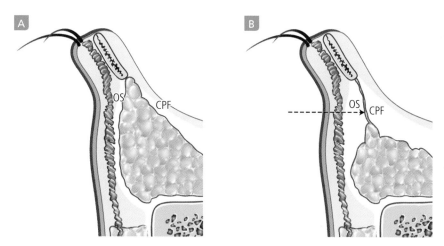

FIGURE 6-18 • **A.** Prior to fat excision. **B.** After fat excision. Excessive excision of orbital fat can allow for direct contact and subsequent adhesion between the capsulopalpebral fascia (CPF) and orbital septum (OS). This can allow for contracture of orbital septum result in decreased elasticity of the capsulopalpebral fascia. Arrow designates the adhesion between the orbital septum and capsulopalpebral fascia.

transfer the post-inflammatory contraction of the septum to the capsulopalpebral fascia, which results in eyelid retraction (FIGURE 6-18).

Fat transposition to the anterior lamella

At times, the nasojugal fold can be very definite and sharp. In such cases, the precision with which the fat is repositioned is a critical matter. Reposition of the fat to the anterior lamella helps to increase this precision. Because the anterior lamella is elevated after midface lift, it is better to fixate the orbital fat to the moving tissue than to the periosteum.

The nasojugal fold coincides with the upper border of cheek fat and also with the border between the preseptal portion and preorbital portion of the orbicularis oculi muscle, all of which belong to the anterior lamella (FIGURE 6-19).

As described above, the supraperiosteal dissection is performed below the orbital rim. Manual compression of the anterior lamella decreases the edema temporarily and allows for palpation of thickness transition at the lid-cheek junction. If the nasojugal fold is visible, a parallel line can be drawn 4-5 mm below the fold. A needle can be inserted through this line to designate the internal location, where the fat can be sutured to the orbicularis muscle with precision.

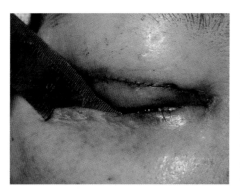

FIGURE 6-19 • Insertion of the ruler between anterior and posterior flaps do not improve the nasojugal fold. However, filling in the same space with gauze demonstrates marked improvement, which suggest that the problem is in the anterior flap.

Transconjunctival fat excision and fat transposition

Transconjunctival fat excision and fat transposition are procedures indicated for excessive laxity of skin and simple pseudoherniation of the orbital fat or nasojugal fold without skin laxity. It can also be used in conjunction with laser therapy to address the fat bulge and lax skin. This transconjunctival approach has also been adopted for midface lift. This approach is favored for avoiding a visible scar. In comparison to the transcutaneous approach, the transconjunctival approach tends to avoid injury to the nerve fibers supplying the pretarsal orbicularis muscle and also minimizes the trauma to anterior lamella and the postoperative scar contracture.

Fat excision

The pseudoherniation of the orbital fat is more prominent in the recumbent position than in the supine position. Therefore, the lower eyelid bulge should be evaluated in the sitting position during the operation. If such a position change is difficult during the operation, the fat bulging can be simulated with manual pressure on the globe while the patient is supine.

Prior to the operation, the fat bulge is evaluated in the sitting position. It may be present in the medial side, or found also in the lateral compartment. Any asymmetry in bulging is committed to memory as well. Once the evaluation is complete, topical anesthetic drops are applied to the conjunctiva, which is subsequently injected with local anesthetics.

Transconjunctival approaches can be divided into preseptal and retroseptal dissection. The preseptal dissection commences with a 10-mm incision placed 1-2 mm below the tarsal plate (5-6 mm inferior to the lower eyelid margin). The dissection

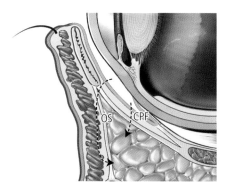

FIGURE 6-20 • The preseptal and retroseptal routes to access the orbital fat.
OS: orbital septum, CPF: Capsulopalpebral fascia.

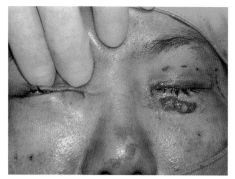

FIGURE 6-21 • Intraoperative photograph of fat excision.
The orbital fat has been excised from the left lower eyelid. The pseudoherniation is demonstrated on the right side by the manipulation of globe.

is carried between the conjunctiva and the orbicularis muscle, down to the inferior orbital rim. At the inferior orbital rim, a 1-cm incision is placed on the periosteum, through which the fat is manually herniated by pressure on the globe. The fat is excised using electrocautery. The retroseptal dissection begins with an incision on the orbital septum 5-6 mm below the tarsal plate. The capsulopalpebral fascia is opened, through which the fat is approached towards the inferior orbital rim and excised **(FIGURE 6-20)**.

Inexperienced operators may experience difficulty in finding the orbital fat. The most foolproof method is to dissect directly to the inferior orbital rim and find the orbital fat just inside the orbital rim.

To evaluate whether the amount of an excision is adequate, manual pressure is applied to temporarily drive away the edema. The lower eyelid is examined with the patient in sitting position. If the sitting position is difficult for the patient, the globe can be pressed to simulate the fat bulging. The operator must become familiar with the approximate amount of manual pressure required to simulate fat bulging, prior to the operation **(FIGURE 6-21)**.

After excision of the fat, the conjunctiva is left to close on its own (secondary intention).

Usually, simple excision of the orbital fat is satisfactory, if the lower eyelid skin is relatively taut. It can even improve the appearance of nasojugal fold. After the 3rd decade of life, the skin becomes lax and begins to wrinkle. In patients with laxity of skin, simple excision of fat can often worsen the appearance of nasojugal fold. Also, excessive excision of fat can result in depression of the area, which was previously bulging.

Transconjunctival fat transposition

The nasojugal fold is demarcated, and a parallel line is drawn 5 mm below the nasojugal fold, to where the fat will be transposed. Anesthetic eye drops are instilled, and local anesthetic is injected into the conjunctiva. A 1.5-cm incision is made on the conjunctiva, and the pretarsal dissection is performed between the orbicularis oculi muscle and the orbital septum, down to the inferior orbital rim. The orbital retaining ligament is divided, and the dissection is carried in either the subperiosteal and supraperiosteal plane. The subperiosteal plane is accessed by opening the periosteum. The supraperiosteal dissection is performed above the levator labii superioris. The medial portion of orbicularis oculi adheres to the orbital rim rather tightly, which makes for difficult dissection. The central portion of the muscle has an indirect connection to the orbital rim, via the orbital retaining ligament, and is easier to dissect.

Through the divided septum, the fat is withdrawn. At times, the septum may be stretched such that it is possible to avoid incising the septum and to mobilize the septum along with the fat. When manipulating the fat, the operator must take care not to injure the inferior oblique muscle, which divided the orbital fat into medial and central fat pad. The inferior oblique muscle is not likely to become traumatized if the operation is carried outside of the orbital rim.

The fat is mobilized using a long double-arm suture, which is driven through the fat and out the skin below the orbicularis muscle at 3 to 4 places. The pull-out sutures are taken out after 4 days. At this time, the important points are 1) mobilization of the fat from surrounding connective tissue (FIGURE 6-22), 2) atraumatic handling of the fat to minimize fat resorption, 3) the medial space to which the fat is transposed must be dissected adequately, as the orbicularis oculi muscle adheres tightly to the orbital rim. 4) When fastening the fat to the anterior lamella, the position at which the suture pierces the orbicularis muscle is important. This should be located 0.5 cm inferior to the nasojugal fold and 1.0 cm inferior to the orbital rim. The location at which the suture exits the skin is not that important. The bolster

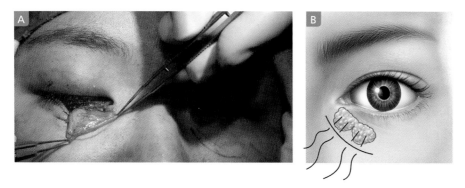

FIGURE 6-22 • **A.** The orbital fat is extracted from the orbital septum. On the left side, the location for fat transposition is marked 5-mm below the nasojugal fold. **B.** An illustration of transposed fat.

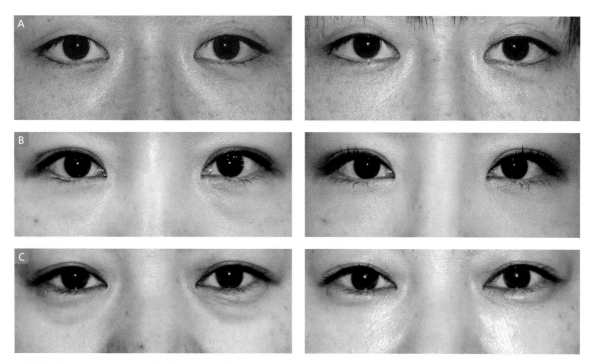

FIGURE 6-23 • Transconjunctival fat transposition.
Preoperative and postoperative photograph.

suture is tied over thick pieces of duoderm. Microfoam is used as a skin splint. The conjunctival wound is approximated and sutured using 7-0 PDS with knots buried.

Lifting the sub-orbicularis oculi fat and the orbicularis oculi muscle (FIGURE 6-24)

The sub-orbicularis oculi fat (SOOF) lift is effective for infraorbital hollowness, caused by deflation and descent of the midfacial fat, and elevates and smooths the lid-cheek junction. It is also helpful in correcting the nasojugal fold and palpebro-malar fold.

In the case of lower lid retraction, SOOF lift alone may not be enough to supplement the lack of skin. In such cases, the orbicularis muscle can be lifted with the rest of the anterior lamella. Structures adjacent to skin must be elevated together in order to augment the eyelid skin.

Upon dissection of the midface, the central portion of the SOOF is pulled to the orbital rim. If either the orbital rim or the SOOF appears friable, the suture can be

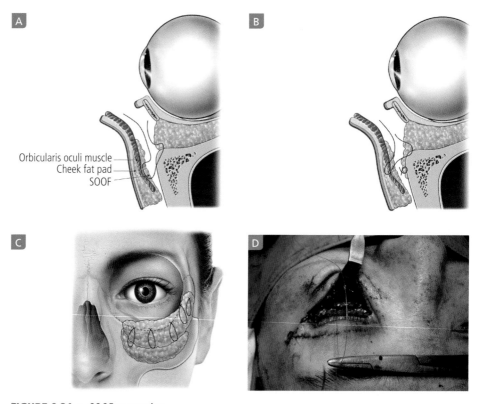

FIGURE 6-24 • SOOF suspension.
The orbicularis muscle and the SOOF are elevated together. If the tissue is too loose, the suture can be looped in the tissue prior to knot tying. **A.** SOOF elevation. **B.** Fat transposition and SOOF elevation. **C.** SOOF elevation, preoperative and postoperative photographs. **D.** Intraoperative photograph of simultaneous fixation of the SOOF and orbicularis muscle to the orbital rim.

driven twice through either or both of the tissues. Additionally, orbicularis suspension is made in the lateral canthal area.

The sub-orbicularis oculi fat is fixated to points medial and lateral to the infra-orbital nerve bundle. The needle is driven through the orbital rim from inside the orbital wall to the outside. This is because the arcus marginalis is a secure anchor that is formed between the periosteum and the septal thickening.

The bottom of orbicularis oculi muscle corresponds to the inferior arc, and fixation of SOOF and orbicularis muscle are elevated and fixed to the orbital rim. To address lagophthalmos from lack of skin, the midface lift is more effective with thinner flaps. If a single fixation appears insecure, the suture can be driven twice through either or both of SOOF and periosteum. If the periosteum appears friable, a hole can be drilled in the orbital rim to be used as an anchor.

Canthal anchoring

This procedure fixates the tarso-ligamentous sling to the orbital rim, which stabilizes the shape and position of the lower lid **(FIGURE 6-26)**.

Indication

- Lower eyelid laxity.
- Exophthalmos
- Lower lid ectropion, retraction
- Prevention of postoperative lower lid malposition due to wound contraction and edema.

Various kinds of lateral canthal anchoring

- Orbicularis oculi muscle canthal anhoring
- Superficial canthal anchoring
- Lateral retinaculum suspension
- Deep canthal tendon anchoring
- Tarsal canthal anchoring, tarsal strip procedure

The choice of operative method depends on the degree of lower lid laxity or exophthalmos. Mild cases can be addressed by pretarsal orbicularis oculi canthal

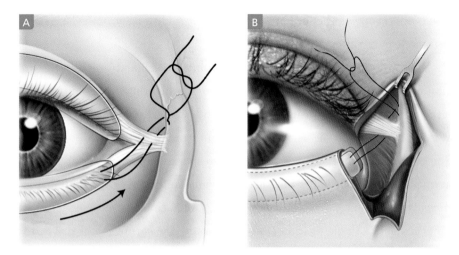

FIGURE 6-25 • **A.** Canthopexy (tarsal suspension, lateral canthal tendon plication, transcanthal canthopexy, OOM canthopexy). **B.** Tarsal strip canthoplasty.

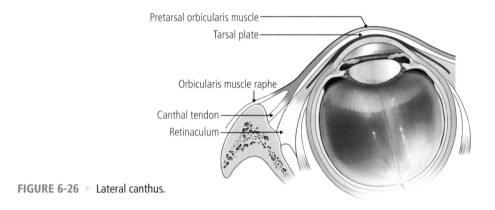

Pretarsal orbicularis muscle
Tarsal plate
Orbicularis muscle raphe
Canthal tendon
Retinaculum

FIGURE 6-26 • Lateral canthus.

anchoring, superficial canthal anchoring, or lateral retinacular suspension. Moderate-to-severe cases require canthal anchoring using the lateral canthal ligament or the lateral portion of the tarsal plate. If the lower eyelid laxity or the exophthalmos is not severe, the lateral canthus is not divided but just fixated without cantholysis (canthopexy). Canthoplasty is performed with horizontal lengthening for severe laxity, by the division of inferior crus of lateral canthal tendon (cantholysis) and refixation (canthoplasty) **(FIGURE 6-25)**.

The most important issue for canthal anchoring (canthopexy or canthoplasty) is selecting the method that provides the most secure fixation in any given case. Secure fixations require the avoidance of suture cheese-wiring through the tissue

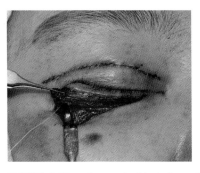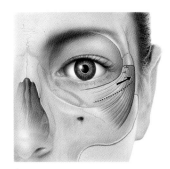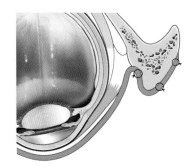

FIGURE 6-27 • Pretarsal orbicularis canthopexy.
The pretarsal orbicularis muscle is fixated to the orbital rim or to the inner surface of the lateral orbital rim.

and the formation of definite adhesion between tissues. Even if the suture is non-absorbable, the eyelid laxity will return without secure adhesion between connective tissues. To create a secure fixation, the operator must understand the advantages and disadvantages of various canthal-anchoring procedures and find the appropriate indicates for each. The fat or orbicularis oculi muscle should be kept out of the way between the tissues that must undergo adhesion. This is because adhesions form between tissues in direct contact with each other. The height and location of fixation is important above all else, and the suture must not be tied with undue force.

Anatomically, the lateral canthal tendon consists of superficial canthal tendon and deep canthal tendon. The former inserts into the anterior surface of the orbital rim **(FIGURE 6-27)**. The latter connects to the Whitnall's tubercle 3-4 mm from the tarsal plate and the orbital rim.

Canthal anchoring can stabilize the shape and position of the lower lid by a relatively atraumatic orbicularis oculi canthopexy to prevent malposition of lower eyelid in patients without much lid laxity **(FIGURE 6-27)**. Connecting the orbicularis oculi muscle to the orbital rim (superficial canthal anchoring method) or by connecting the tarsal plate, the canthal tendon, or the retinaculum to the Whitnall's tubercle that is 2-3 mm inside the lateral orbital rim (deep canthal anchoring method). In severe exophthalmos, the tarsal plate can be fixed to the orbital rim to avoid deep fixation. For lower lid laxity or for correction of lid retraction or ectropion, canthal tendon is fixated to the periosteum about 3 mm inward from the lateral orbital rim. The tissues are fixated using 5-0 Ethibond or Mersilene suture with double-arm needles.

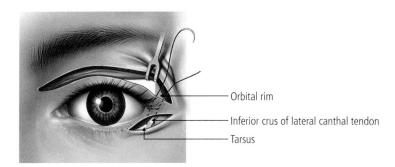

Orbital rim

Inferior crus of lateral canthal tendon

Tarsus

FIGURE 6-28 • Lateral retinaculum suspension: The retinaculum is passed through the canthus and secured to the lateral orbital tubercle.

The suture is tied without undue tension.

Pretarsal orbicularis canthopexy (FIGURE 6-27)

Among various canthopexy methods, the pretarsal orbicularis canthopexy is a conservative, relatively atraumatic method that is appropriate for patients without much canthal laxity and for prevention of postoperative lower lid malposition. In this technique, the lateral end of the pretarsal orbicularis muscle is fixated at the orbital rim to the inner surface of the orbital rim. As with other canthopexy methods, the lower eyelid should have enough laxity for 1-2 mm on distraction test. The advantage of this method is that there is no direct trauma to the lateral canthal ligament.

Lateral retinaculum suspension (FIGURE 6-28)

Lateral retinaculum can be synonymous with lateral canthus but can also refer to the structure surrounding the canthal tendon and attaches to the lateral orbital tubercle (Whitnall's tubercle).

The anatomy of lateral retinaculum (FIGURE 6-29)

(Lateral canthal tendon)

The lateral horn of levator aponeurosis

Whitnall's ligament

Inferior suspensory ligament (Lockwood ligament)

Check ligament of lateral rectus muscle

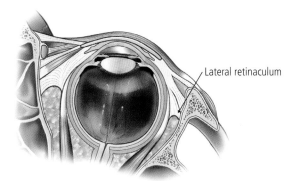

FIGURE 6-29 • Lateral retinaculum.

The location for fixation

The lateral portion of tarsus and the pretarsal oculi muscle are simultaneously fixed to a point just superior to the lateral orbital tubercle. In 3-dimensions, the fixation location can be considered:

1. Vertical – height
2. Anterior/posterior – inner distance from the lateral orbital rim
3. Horizontal – adjusted by the tension placed by the fixation

Fixations are more secure when incorporating both tarsal plate and the canthal tendon (transcanthal).

For severe eyelid laxity (greater than 6 mm on eyelid distraction test) the lower eyelid can be shortened by wedge resection (canthoplasty). If the amount of resection is same between the skin and tarsal tissue, the skin will be under too much tension after closure, and the resection should be not be a rectangle but a wedge in shape. No more than 2-to-3 mm of the lower eyelid should be resected, and the shortened eyelid should have about 1-to-2 mm of distraction. If the eyelid is shortened excessively, the horizontal tension can cause the eyelid to assume a lower position or higher position in the case of enophthalmos.

At times, the wedge resection can be performed first. At others, the canthal anchoring is performed, and the wedge resection is performed if there is redundancy of the lower eyelid, which results in buckling towards the lateral canthus **(FIGURE 6-31B)**.

The location for canthal fixation varies depending on the degree of

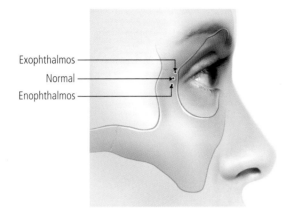

Exophthalmos

Normal

Enophthalmos

FIGURE 6-30 • Anchoring point according to exophthal-metry.

The inferior margin of the pupil is used as the reference point in neutral globe protrusion.

enophthalmos-exophthalmos. In most cases, the lateral canthus is fixed to the level of inferior margin of the pupil. However, in the presence of exophthalmos, the canthus is fixated in a high and superficial location on the orbital rim. Too high of a canthal fixation can result in severe positive canthal tilt (i.e. Madame Butterfly eyes), which can narrow the palpebral fissure. In the case of enophthalmos, the canthus should be fixated at a point that is lower and deeper than the usual fixation point (FIGURE 6-30). If the fixation is too high, the eyes appear 'squinty', whereas too shallow of a fixation can result in distracted eyelid. If the canthal tendon is to be fixated deeper into the orbital wall, a double-arm suture should be used from within and passed outward to ensure a secure fixation. If the periosteum is friable during a secondary operation, an anchoring hole can be drilled in the orbital rim, through which a suture is passed from within the orbit to outside. The suture is then fixated to the periosteum or to the temporal fascia. Upon fixation, the palpebral fissure and the canthal angle should be evaluated for symmetry in the sitting position. A tensionless fixation is important for decreasing the risk of lid laxity relapse.

The degree of globe protrusion is evaluated using Hertel exophthalmometer. A distance of 15-to-18 mm is considered to be within normal range. More than 18 mm of distance is defined to be exophthalmia, whereas less than 15 mm of distance is considered enophthalmia.

In order to maintain proper contact between the globe and the lower eyelid, the upper border of the tarsus should be secured deep in the orbital rim. The double-arm needle is used such that the upper arm takes a bigger bite of the tarsal plate, without twisting the plate. The fixation must be made with minimal tension. The

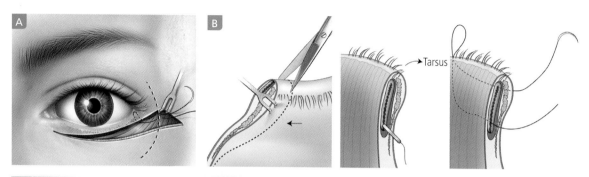

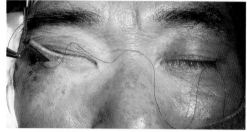

FIGURE 6-31 ● High fixation of the tarsal plate.
A. Canthopexy. The tarsal plate is first closed using a horizontal mattress suture. A stab incision is placed just on the side of the grey line, through which the needle is passed. **B.** Canthoplasty. The suture is passed from below to the top of the tarsal plate. This method provides a secure fixation because it incorporates a large portion of the tarsal plate.

fixation should be conducive to the formation of adhesion, for the new canthal position to be secure.

Summary

Exophthalmos

1. Upward and anterior anchoring
2. No horizontal shortening
3. Retractor release with of without spacer graft
4. Less tension

Enophthalmos

1. Deep and posterior anchoring
2. Downward fixation
3. Intensive tie

Generally, the lower eyelid is easier to fixate higher than lower. Because of this, the author prefers to fixate the lower portion of tarsal plate. If the ectropion is severe, however, fixation of the upper portion of tarsal plate is helpful in controlling the ectropion **(FIGURE 6-31)**.

Pretarsal orbicularis oculi muscle canthopexy

Among the various canthal anchoring technique, this method is relatively conservative and atraumatic one . it can be used in the case of no or little canthal laxity and for prevention of postoperative eyelid malposition. Operation technique is fixation of the lateral end of pretarsal oculi muscle to the inside of orbital rim periosteum. After operation, distraction amount is within 1-3 mm, that is the difference from the orbicularis oculi suspension technique. Advantages of this technique is there is no direct trauma of lateral cantus. This technique can not be used for the lateral canthal laxity **(FIGURE 6-27)**.

High fixation of the tarsal plate

Canthopexy method

A small stab incision is made in the conjunctiva near the mucosal-skin transition of lateral canthal angle. A 4-0 Prolene or PDS suture is passed through this point and then the tarsal plate. To avoid cheese-wiring, a 7-0 nylon can be placed as a locking suture over the 4-0 suture, or the 4-0 suture can be passed once through the tarsal plate and then through the stab incision above the grey line **(FIGURE 6-31A)**.

Canthoplasty method

On the resected surface of lower eyelid, the needle is driven through the tarsal plate from below to above and secured on the periosteum of the deep aspect of the lateral orbital rim. The higher arm of the suture should be placed high, and the lower arm of the suture must be placed low – such that the same offset distance is maintained on both the tarsal plate and the periosteum. This prevents twisting of the tarsal plate. In most situations, a wedge section of 2-3 mm is resected off the lower eyelid and tarsal plate. The resected edges must be accurately re-approximated at the time of closure to avoid blunting of the canthal angle. To allow the upper eyelid to slightly rest on top of the lower eyelid, the grey line of the upper eyelid is sutured onto the grey line of the lower eyelid such that the upper margin is anterior to the lower margin.

The fixation point on the orbital rim (i.e. height and depth) must vary according to the degree of exophthalmos. In East Asian patients, there is a tendency for a slight positive canthal tilt. As such, it is important to make sure the fixation is not too

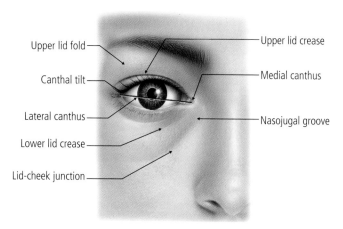

FIGURE 6-32 • The degree and tilt of the canthal line.

Per anthropometry in Korean population, the usual range of canthal tilt ranges from 5 to 10 degrees. Assuming a palpebral fissure width of 30 mm, this translates to a lateral canthus that is 2.6 to 5.3 mm higher than the medial canthus. For reference, a 2-mm of canthal height difference equates to a canthal tilt of 3.8 degrees, with a 4-mm height difference equating to 7.6 degrees.

high (i.e. madame butterfly eye). The line connecting the medial canthus and the lateral canthus defines the canthal tilt, which varies according to age, sex, and across ethnicities. Compared to Caucasian patients, East Asian patients tend to have a higher canthal tilt, with a canthal tilt of 5-10 degrees and the lateral canthus about 3-5 mm higher than the medial canthus (**FIGURE 6-32**).

The strength with which the lower eyelid wraps the anterior surface of the eye is important. In exophthalmos, greater tension across the lower eyelid results in a lower position. In enophthalmos, greater tension in the lower eyelid results in a higher position. To account for lowered eyelid height in the postoperative period, the canthus must be anchored such that the lower eyelid margin covers 1-2 mm of the corneal limbus, with a slight degree of canthal tilt. In primary operations, mild overcorrection to cover the corneal limbus is adequate (1-mm overlap), whereas the overcorrection must be commensurate (2-mm of limbus coverage) with the decreased elasticity of lower eyelid in secondary operations.

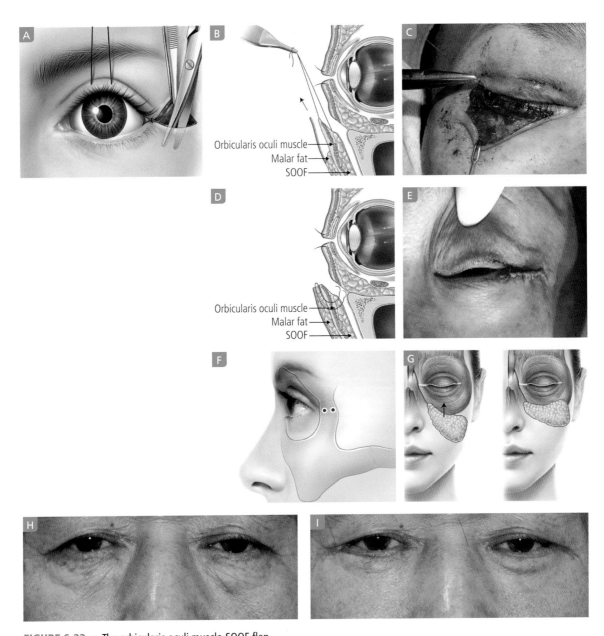

FIGURE 6-33 • The orbicularis oculi muscle-SOOF flap.
A, B, C. When elevating the orbicularis muscle, the sub-orbicularis oculi fat and the malar fat (cheek fat) are also elevated. **D.** orbicularis oculi muscle suspension. **E.** SOOF and malar fat before and after the suspension. **F.** Pre/postoperative photographs of a patient who underwent the procedure.

Orbicularis oculi muscle suspension (FIGURE 6-33)

The preseptal orbicularis muscle flap is fixated with more than two suspension sutures: 1) the lateral orbicularis muscle flap is suspended to the lateral orbital periosteum or the deep temporal fascia, and 2) just the medial portion of the orbicularis muscle flap is suspended to the lateral orbital rim. When suspending the orbicularis muscle, the separation of orbicularis muscle flap by subcutaneous dissection is useful in elevating the lower eyelid and avoiding skin depression (FIGURE 6-33C). However, subcutaneous dissection is traumatic to the skin and therefore should be minimized to lower the risk of skin dimpling. When fixating the orbicularis muscle to the periosteum, it is important to pull the eyelid up with adequate tension. However, the suture should not be tied too tightly because the muscle is weak against pressure. The author finds that the orbicularis oculi muscle is too weak to be suspended alone and incorporates SOOF into the suspension.

The advantages of this technique are that it lifts the skin and the SOOF, the latter of which corrects the infraorbital hollowness (FIGURE 6-33E). It also bolsters the lower eyelid mechanism and resists the pseudoherniation of orbital fat. Both the malar fat pad and cheek fat are lifted (FIGURE 6-33B), which improves the appearance of the lid-cheek junction. Although it belongs to the anterior lamella, the SOOF-orbicularis muscle flap buttresses and supports the lateral canthal tendon (orbicularis oculi muscle sling effect). The method performs a variety of functions and is a very valuable procedure.

Various functions of orbicularis oculi muscle suspension

- Midface lift
- Correction of the nasojugal fold and palpebromalar fold
- Correction of infraorbital hollowness
- Augmentation of the skin shortage
- Smoothing of the malar area
- Blending of the lid-cheek junction and malar crescent

Thus far, the operation can be applied to uncomplicated primary operations as well as for patients with lower lid malposition (i.e. scleral show or ectropion).

Excision of skin and pretarsal orbicularis muscle

Skin excision should be conservative. Preservation of the lower lid skin is especially important for midface lift or for those secondary operations with ectropion or scleral show. In the latter group of patients, the lower lid margin may become lower by 1-1.5 mm in the postoperative period, and the adequate amount of skin should be left alone to account for this change. Intraoperatively, the amount of skin to be excised is evaluated by having the patient in a sitting position and in primary gaze. The patient is instructed to gently open the mouth. The skin is pulled superiorly, and vertical incisions are made on the skin flap, which serve to compartmentalize the amount of skin excision along the length of the eyelid (FIGURE 6-34).

The orbicularis oculi muscle should not be excised as much as the skin is excised. The pretarsal OOM performs an important role in maintaining the natural shape of the lower eyelid and should not be excised except for hypertrophy of the orbicularis oculi muscle. Pretarsal fullness has been discussed at length already. As such, the

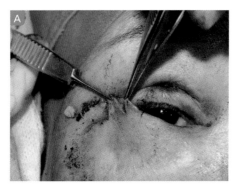
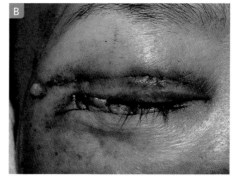
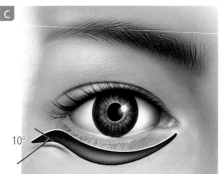

FIGURE 6-34 • **A.** Vertical incisions are made to compartmentalize the amount of skin to be excised. **B.** The lower flap is divided by 4 vertical incisions along the length of the eyelid. **C.** The main horizontal incision should have a 10 degree of deflection towards the inferolateral direction.

following will serve as a brief reminder. The pretarsal fullness is created by covering the pretarsal orbicularis oculi muscle with the preseptal orbicularis muscle. Pretarsal flatness or depression can be considered as yet another phenomenon of the aging process. It can be caused by decrease in the tonicity of the orbicularis muscle and the descent of the pretarsal structure, which gives the appearance of standoffish countenance. Conversely, a person with pretarsal fullness appears youthful and approachable. Restoration of pretarsal fullness requires a) bunching of the pretarsal orbicularis muscle and b) covering of this pretarsal orbicularis muscle with the preseptal orbicularis muscle from the lower flap. The pretarsal fullness should be located as close to the lower eyelid margin as possible. The pretarsal portion of the muscle is very important for this purpose and should be preserved as much as possible. Also, the operator must understand that the pretarsal fullness requires adequate skin laxity to match the volume of muscle underneath.

Beyond the lateral canthus, the incision is extended to account for the amount of skin excision. The extension angle is most appropriate at approximately 10 degrees **(FIGURE 6-34C)**.

The wound is closed using quilted suture to minimize the dead space in the lateral portion. The closed skin must be everted along the whole incision to minimize the risk of depressed scar.

Frost sutures or tarsorrhaphy may be necessary to pull up the lower eyelid, if ectropion persist after skin closure or if the orbicularis muscle is weak.

The skin is splinted using Microfoam dressing. The lower eyelid skin is maximally stretched prior to applying the foam, which boosts the lower eyelid margin by a 1 mm **(FIGURE 6-35)**.

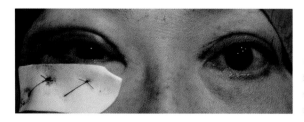

FIGURE 6-35 • The lower eyelid is splinted. Quilting suture is placed on top of the Microfoam to obliterate any dead space and prevent postoperative edema.

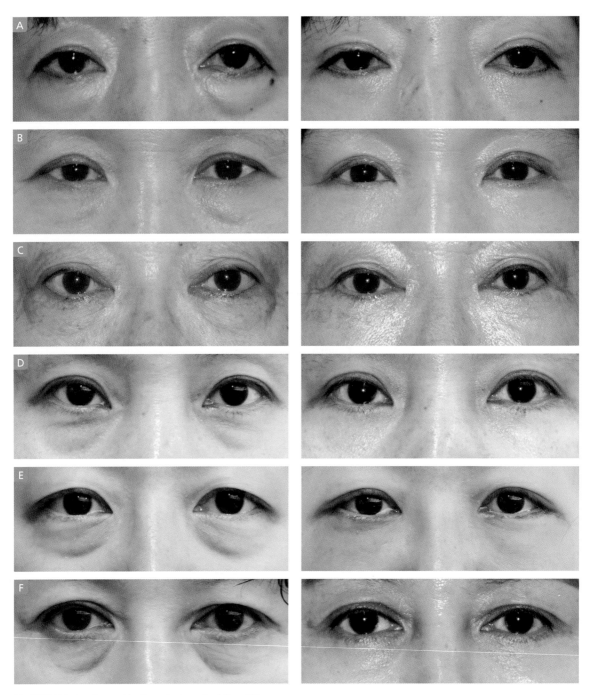

FIGURE 6-36 • Lower blepharoplasty and midface lift.

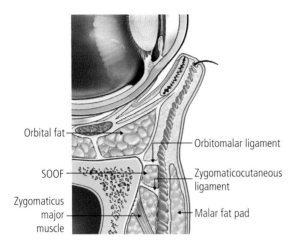

Orbital fat
SOOF
Zygomaticus major muscle

Orbitomalar ligament
Zygomaticocutaneous ligament
Malar fat pad

FIGURE 6-37 • Periorbital fat.

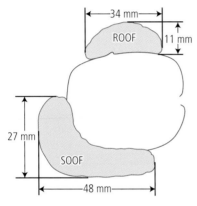

FIGURE 6-38 • Retro-orbicularis oculi fat and sub-orbicularis oculi fat.

Crescent of ROOF is mostly above supraorbital rim, yet also a few millimeters below rim. Horizontal length of ROOF is 34 mm and vertical height 11 mm. Hockey stick-shaped head of SOOF is mostly below lower orbital rim, yet also a few millimeters over inferolateral orbital rim. Horizontal length is 48 mm and vertical height 27 mm.

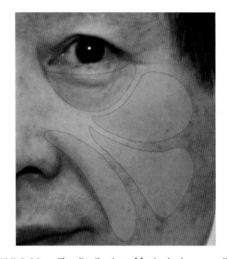

FIGURE 6-39 • The distribution of fat in the lower eyelid and the midface.

PERIORBITAL FAT

The periorbital fat are discussed in sections. Some of the operations have already been discussed above and will only be summarized here.

The fat around the lower eyelid can be divided into 3 sections.

- Orbital fat **(FIGURE 6-37)**
- Sub-orbicularis oculi fat **(FIGURE 6-38)**
- Subcutaneous fat (malar fat and cheek fat) **(FIGURE 6-39)**

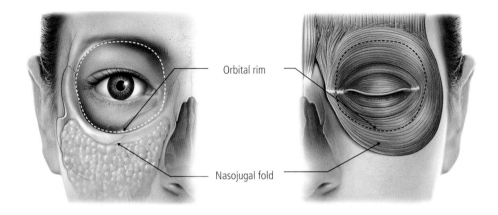

Orbital rim

Nasojugal fold

FIGURE 6-40 • The upper border of cheek fat coincides with the nasojugal fold and palpebromalar fold. It is also the border between the preseptal and preorbital portions of the orbicularis muscle.

Correlations between facial aging and changes in fat tissue

Nasojugal fold and palpebromalar fold

- Coincides with the lower border of pseudoherniated orbital fat
- Depression from SOOF descent
- The upper border of cheek fat

Malar crescent

- Border of malar fat

Inferior orbital hollowness

- Descent of SOOF

Nasolabial fold

- Descent of cheek fat

Lower blepharoplasty with manipulation of periorbital fat

Orbital fat

Simple excision. Discussed above.

This method decreases the fat bulging. It may or may not improve the nasojugal fold **(FIGURE 6-43)**. Excessive excision of the orbital fat can not only cause sunken eyelid but can also contribute to enophthalmos and eyeball downward displacement. Traumatic inflammation of the orbital fat can lead to the formation of adhesion between the septum and the retractor. Contraction of the septum can lead to lower eyelid descent.

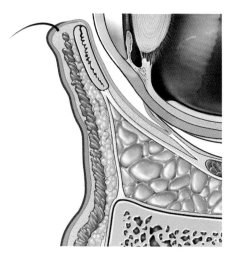

FIGURE 6-41 • Location of micro fat transfer.
Between orbicularis oculi muscle and periosteum and between orbicularis oculi muscle and the septum.

Micro fat injection

The fat is injected along the nasojugal fold and infraorbital hollowness. This method can mask slight bulging of the orbital fat.

Operative detail

To increase the survival rate of fat cells, the liposuction is performed at the lowest level of vacuum through a 12 gauge. The author prefers to obtain micro fat graft from the thigh or the medial portion of the knee over that obtained from the abdomen. The fat from the lower extremity is less fibrous and suppler with lower tissue-particulate volume.

The fat injection is performed with the patient in sitting position because the

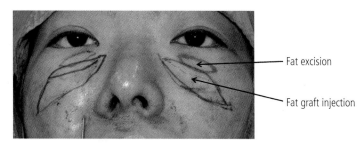

Fat excision

Fat graft injection

FIGURE 6-42 • Micro fat transfer technique.
The injection is performed in a sitting position.

shape and location of bulging and depression changes with position. In the supine position, the fat will be injected in a more superior position, compared to that injected in the sitting position. Also, it is important to identify any fat bulging or soft tissue irregularities that occur with specific facial expressions.

Just inferior to the orbital rim, the fat should be injected in the deep plane – just superficial to the periosteum – to avoid clumping of the fat in the skin. Above the orbital rim, the micro fat should be injected in multiple layers. One milliliter (1 ml) of the fat is injected over 40 micro-aliquots in varying directions and layers to avoid causing skin irregularity and to increase survival rate of fat cells. The amount of fat injection is 1.5 times the amount of sunken volume – an overcorrection to account for fat resorption. Cool compression is applied after the transfer.

Excision of orbital fat with subsequent micro fat transfer (FIGURE 6-44)

The bulging orbit fat is excised, and the micro fat is injected into the depressed

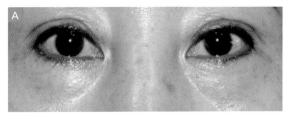
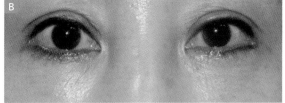

FIGURE 6-43 • Before and after excision of orbital fat.

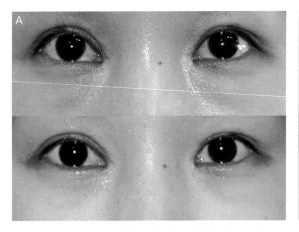
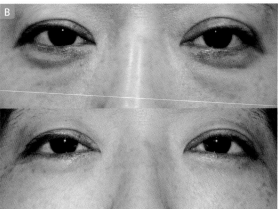

FIGURE 6-44 • Fat excision and micro fat injection to the nasojugal fold.

areas – nasojugal fold and infraorbital hollowness. The fat is injected in multiple planes – supraperiosteal, sub-orbicularis oculi fat, orbicularis muscle, and subcutaneous plane. Wherever the layer is thin (e.g. subcutaneous layer), the micro fat is injected in extremely small quantities to avoid creating surface irregularities.

Fat transposition (FIGURE 6-45)

As discussed previously, the bulging fat is decreased. The space between the orbicularis muscle and the periosteum is dissected. The orbital fat is moved 4-5 mm below the upper border of cheek fat – below the orbitomalar ligament – to augment the nasojugal fold.

SOOF

Sub-orbicularis oculi fat is mobilized to lift the lid-cheek junction and augment the infraorbital hollowness.

Cheek fat

Cheek fat is in the subcutaneous layer. Orbicularis oculi suspension lift can bring up the cheek fat and malar fat. This improves the malar crescent and nasolabial fold.

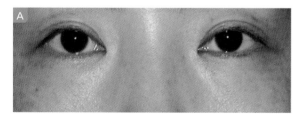
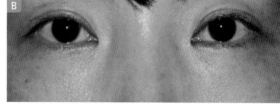

FIGURE 6-45 ● Orbital fat transposition.

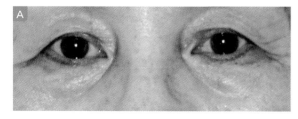
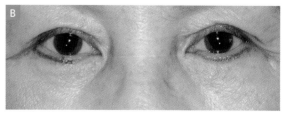

FIGURE 6-46 ● Orbital fat transposition and SOOF elevation.

LOWER LID RETRACTION

A common yet severe complication of lower blepharoplasty is lid retraction. This malposition of lower eyelid includes lateral canthal rounding, scleral show, distraction and cicatrical ectropion. At times, scleral show without ectropion is also considered to be lid retraction as well.

Primary lower lid malposition is frequently observed in the elderly population, and can be caused by tarsoligament laxity or disinsertion or by hypotonicity of the orbicularis muscle. Secondary lid malpositions are generally caused by periorbital cicatrical forces from a previous operation. Secondary retractions can also be caused by excessive excision of skin or orbicularis muscle or by cicatrical contraction from postoperative inflammatory changes to the orbital septum. Clinically, severe hematoma is often followed by lid retraction. Even if the hematoma is removed early, traces of inflammatory cytokines are left in the orbicularis muscle, orbital septum, or capsulopalpebral fascia, which leads to severe cicatrical contracture. This phenomenon can be observed for fat injections around the orbital septum in open blepharoplasty. Because of this, presence of hematoma requires not only re-exploration to remove the hematoma itself but also to perform preventative measures against retraction.

The degree of lid malposition is evaluated by the distance between the corneal limbus and the lower eyelid margin. Normally, the eyelid margin lies at the lower limbus or covers about 1 mm of the limbus **(FIGURE 6-47)**. The amount of scleral show is evaluated measured medially, centrally, and laterally.

In addition to the aesthetic problem, eyelid retraction can lead to epiphora, blurred vision, foreign body sensation, decreased visual acuity, light sensitivity, xerophthalmia, and even exposure keratitis.

The xerophthalmia from eyelid retraction is caused by the inability of the lower

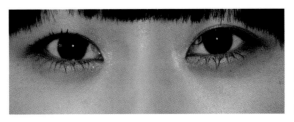

FIGURE 6-47 • In the right eye, the eyelid crease is much fainter from the ptosis.

eyelid to oppose or hug the anterior surface of the globe. This separation leads to the keratinization of the orifice of the meibomian (tarsal) gland near the posterior border of the mucocutaneous junction of the lower lid. The significant decrease in the lipid secretion allows accelerated evaporation of the aqueous tear. However, the keratinization process can be reversed if the retraction is corrected. In addition, ectropion of the medial eyelid can lead to keratinization of the lacrimal punctum, leading to obstruction of the outflow. Weakness of the orbicularis muscle can also aggravate the process by the decrease in the lacrimal pump.

A wide variety of procedures are performed to correct eyelid retraction.

Prior to any given procedure, the operator must ascertain whether the retraction is limited to the anterior lamella, the posterior lamella, or a combination of both.

In the case of excessive skin excision, the problem is most likely in the anterior lamella. However, the problem could also be caused by posterior lamella issues (e.g. hematoma or cicatrical contraction). In many cases, the retraction may be caused by a problem in a single layer, which is transferred to the other layer during the redraping process.

Lower eyelid retraction can be evaluated with forced elevation test, as reported by McCord et al. and Patipa. Intraoperatively, dissection of the anterior lamella isolates the posterior lamella. If the retraction persists even after dissection, the posterior lamella is contributing to the retraction. The author evaluates lower eyelid retraction by pinching the skin at the inferior orbital rim and pulls it upward. If this maneuver temporarily allows the lower eyelid margin to rise to a normal position without tension, then the problem is exclusive to the anterior lamella. If, however, this "helping hand" does not allow the eyelid margin to rise to a normal level, then the posterior lamella will need to be explored. If the skin has enough laxity and wrinkles, the problem is usually with the posterior lamella.

The most important aspect of correcting lower lid retraction is to lift the eyelid skin with adequate laxity and to prevent the lifted anterior lamella from drooping again. The midface lift allows the eyelid skin to be lifted with redundancy. The re-drooping of eyelid is prevented with canthal anchoring and orbicularis suspension technique. The next important goal is to release any contracture in the middle and posterior lamellae from the inferior border of tarsus to the inferior orbital rim.

Minor ectropion can be addressed with canthoplasty, tarsal strip procedure, wedge resection, or orbicularis muscle suspension. Moderate degree of retraction requires dissection of the cicatrical contracture with conjunction of canthoplasty and/or midface lift (orbicularis muscle suspension). In severe cases, the middle and posterior lamellae must be dissected to release the contractures. Spacer grafts are most likely required. Complete release of the cicatrical contraction is important. Correction of lid retraction is important not only for aesthetics but also for eyelid function.

Retraction from anterior lamella

- Midface lift and orbicularis muscle suspension, canthoplasty
- Skin graft

Retraction from posterior lamella

Retractors such as capsulopalpebral fascia and inferior tarsal muscle are released along with cicatrical contraction in the orbital septum. In severe cases, spacer graft is used to augment the posterior lamella.

When the lower lid laxity is minor and the distraction test is less than 7 mm, canthopexy is appropriate. However, distraction distances greater than 7 mm should be addressed by tarsal strip procedure, wedge resection, canthoplasty. Orbicularis oculi muscle and sub-orbicularis oculi fat should is lifted together. Correction of lid retraction is important not only for aesthetics but also for function (xerophthalmia, exposure keratopathy, chemosis, and decrease visual acuity).

High risk patient

- Exophthalmos
- Malar hypoplasia
- High myopia
- Pre-existing scleral show
- Lid laxity – hypotonia
- Secondary blepharoplasty

In relation to the orbital wall, protrusion of the globe is a negative vector, which is considered to be a risk factor. In addition, lower lid laxity and prior history of blepharoplasty can also be considered to be high risk.

Release of lower lid retractors and spacer graft

As previously discussed, retractions limited to the anterior lamella are addressed using midface lift and skin graft, canthal anchoring, and/or orbicularis oculi suspension.

For retractions of middle-posterior lamellae, the adhesions are released in areas surrounding the orbital septum and the inferior retinaculum (**FIGURE 6-48**). Lysis of the contracted tissues and the inferior retractors (capsulopalpebral fascia) restores 1 mm of eyelid margin height. However, this alone is inadequate in most cases, and the operator must be aware of the fact that these dissected structures may adhere again. In principle, releasing the retractor has a preventative effect, but retractions from posterior lamella can only be corrected by spacer graft.

In addition, the inferior deviation of lower eyelid can become severe from severe exophthalmos and postoperative hematoma. Spacer graft can also be used in such cases. The spacer can be autologous (aponeurosis, sclera, ear cartilage, septal cartilage, palatal mucosa, dermis, or dermofat) or allogeneic (Enduragen, cadaveric aponeurosis, Alloderm, and Lyoplast). The hard palatal mucosa graft has relatively minimal contraction and mild edema. However, the operation is technically challenging, and the donor-site pain is a significant discomfort to the patient. Dermal graft has minimal contraction and has a relatively good survival rate. Dermofat graft is useful for augmenting hollowness in the lower eyelid and also functions as a buttress to the lifted tissues. It is also effective as a buffer to keep the dissected structures separated. Dermal graft can be taken from postauricular area or below the ilium. Dermofat can be taken from below the iliac crest. Alloplastic material tends to cause significant postoperative edema and prolongs the recovery period from increased inflammation.

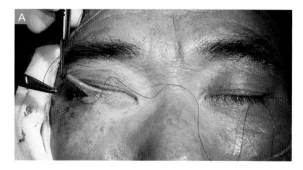
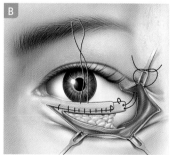

FIGURE 6-48 • Tarsal strip procedure is performed after releasing the retractors and surrounding tissues such as the inferior retinaculum.

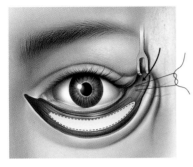
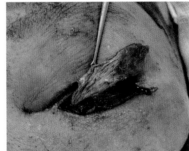
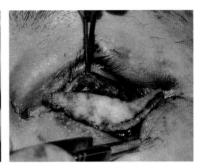

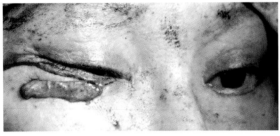

FIGURE 6-49 • Spacer graft. Deep temporal fascia graft. Allogeneic dermal graft. Dermofat graft.

However, it is readily available. Thicker alloplastic materials tend to undergo less contraction but can add too much bulk to the lower eyelid (FIGURE 6-49).

Where the retractors have been release, the orbicularis oculi muscle that has been elevated from the midface procedure can be used as a spacer flap.

The spacer graft is placed in the dissected space after the contracted tissue is completely released and the canthal anchoring is completed. Compared to autologous grafts, allogeneic grafts require twice as much spacing to account for the increased amount of contraction. This, however, must be balanced against the fact that large allogeneic grafts are more likely to elicit inflammatory response. One important consideration in spacer grafting is that of the blood supply to the eyelid margin. With the division of contracted septum, the superior flap of the eyelid becomes a bipedicled flap. However, canthotomy turns this bi-pedicled flap into a flap with a long single pedicle, which should be avoided. Because of this issue, the author releases the surrounding contracted tissue from the conjunctiva without division of the conjunctiva. The spacer graft is laid on top of the intact conjunctiva. Preservation of conjunctiva tends to decrease the risk of inflammatory response even for larger allograft. If the conjunctiva does not cover the graft, inflammation and graft failure are more likely.

Prior to spacer graft placement, the posterior lamella is first released. The canthus

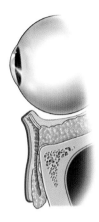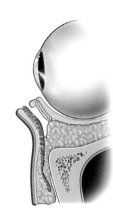

FIGURE 6-50 • Elevation of the lower eyelid. Before and after midface lifting.

is anchored to elevate the lower eyelid, which secures an empty space to be grafted. When accounting for postoperative contraction, this space and the graft must be large. In other words, the spacer graft does not perform the role of elevating the eyelid. Rather, the malpositioned eyelid is restored to the normal physiologic position by releasing the contracted tissue and by canthal anchoring, and the spacer graft is simply a deterrence against further retraction. The spacer grafts can occasionally be used for partial augmentation. However, if the retraction is present along the whole width of the eyelid, the graft should be prepared long enough to reach the lateral canthus.

The author applies to 1 ml of triamcinolone (diluted to 2 mg/ml) to the wound to minimize the risk of contracture that can occur from minor hematoma after midface lift.

Tarsorraphy or Frost suture are performed. Either of the maneuvers immobilizes the lower eyelid and minimizes the postoperative edema. Eyepatch is also applied for the same reason. Application of Microfoam will lead to elevation of the lower eyelid margin. The use of quilting suture on top of Microfoam is useful in preventing edema.

Avoiding failures in correcting eyelid retraction

In the immediate postoperative period following corrective operation, the lower eyelid margin may cover the bottom 1-mm of the corneal limbus and appear successful. However, this eyelid margin can gradually lower until it returns to the retracted position prior to operation, over the course of 3 weeks to 3 months, which is quite a predicament. What is the cause of this recurrence and what can be done to avoid this embarrassment? The challenge to accurately reset the height of the eyelid margin to the desired position is a very attractive proposition for plastic surgeons.

Even the weakest of force can bring about a large change, when this force is constant over a period of time. Dental malocclusion can be corrected with weak but constant pressure of orthodontics. If the force that pulls the lower eyelid down is constant, the operator must consider methods that counteract this force.

The suture must be able to hold the surgical construct together for the 3 months after the operation while the adhesions are continuing to form between tissues. However, the lower tarsal plate is relatively short and thin, and the inferior crus of lateral canthal tendon can be injured easiliy by 4-0 or 5-0 suture needles. Cheese wiring is also a possibility. Unfortunately, these problems are compounded in secondary operations where the tissues are lacking in both volume and elasticity. It is for this reason that tensions must be minimized throughout the newly created lower eyelid construct. A secure fixation does not need to be under tension, but the ideal technique must result in a structure that can withstand minimal yet pervasive forces acting on the lower eyelid. Following are examples of this principle:

To correct lower lid malposition satisfactorily, the following two issues should be considered.

1. The anterior and posterior lamellae of the lower eyelid are sufficiently elevated.
2. The elevated tissues are prevented from descending again.

   - To maximally elevate the lower eyelid, all of the structures tethering the eyelid must be released – anatomic structures including the orbitomalar ligament, zygomatico-cutaneous ligament, and lateral thickening as well as cicatrical contractions from prior operations. The lower eyelid must be fully released prior to anchoring the canthus. At the time of canthal anchoring, bringing up the lower eyelid must be free of any tension.

   - Thicker flap will bring up deep tissues such as preperiosteal fat and SOOF, which has the advantage of addressing the inferior hollowness. However, thicker flaps do not elevate as much of the skin and orbicularis muscle, that is essential for skin recruit. Because of this, the author places the suspension suture relatively superficially when lifting the SOOF to incorporate the orbicularis muscle in the elevation.

- To keep elevated lower eyelid from retracting again, canthal anchoring should be mechanically robust, and the orbicularis suspension should be effective. To tighten a loose clothesline, the ends be wrapped around secure columns (canthal anchoring) as well as decreasing the weight load (SOOF and orbicularis muscle suspension). Here, secure fixation does not equate to tightness of suture but rather a soft fixation that maintains tissues in place with minimum tension. For secure canthal anchoring, the anchoring tissue (tarsus and/or canthal ligament) should be isolated accurately and fixed to proper location on the periosteum for secure adhesion. To incorporate a large portion of the tarsal plate, the suture can be passed into the plate long distance as demonstrated in **FIGURE 6-31**.

- The canthus can be anchored to a hole drilled through the lateral orbital rim. The author prefers to use drilled hole when the canthus must be fixated deep in the orbital wall or the periosteum is friable. Transcanthal canthopexy is another method for deeper fixation. The periosteum is relatively thick on the lateral orbital rim but is less than appropriate for fixation deep in the orbital wall. (Song) The suture must be placed deep for ectropion, severe eyelid laxity, and enophthalmos.- Canthal anchoring is performed such that the eyelid has 1-2 mm of laxity on distraction test.

- Orbicularis suspension technique can be used in conjunction with tarsal canthopexy for enforcement.

- The canthal anchoring is performed to slightly overcorrect the height and depth.

- The tarsal plate is best fixated in the upper portion.

- Any tissue that is weak alone should be incorporated to a more robust tissue such as patch graft.

- Round needles are preferable to cutting needle for minimizing trauma to the tarsal plate, canthal tendon, or the periosteum.

- After fixation, lower lid position is confirmed in sitting position.

- Nylon and PDS sutures are relatively elastic and can stretch. Canthal anchoring sutures should be performed with inelastic sutures such as Mersilene, Ethibond, or wires.

- When a single fixation is not adequate, tissues must be secured with multiple fixations. The orbicularis suspension should be fixated with multiple sutures.

- Spacer graft may be longer to the length of lateral canthal ligament. The volume of spacer graft may be more important than length (e.g. dermofat graft). Spacer grafts functions as buffers and preventive measures against contraction.
- Extra tissues remaining after elevation should be excised as minimally as possible.
- Tarsorrhaphy is effective in stabilizing the lower eyelid position in the post-operative setting. It is maintained for 2 weeks.
- Skin grafts should be considered.

POSTOPERATIVE MANAGEMENT

The patient is instructed to rest for a day and to keep the head elevated (> 45 degrees). Cool compress is applied over the eyes. Antibiotic ointment is applied to the lower eyelid margin and eyeball 2-3 times a day. An eye drop with a combination of antibiotic and steroid is instilled 2-3 times a day as well. The ointment acts as a lubricant and helps to decrease conjunctival edema. Artificial tears may be used for 1 week. Patients are instructed to sleep with the head of bed elevated with a pillows. Steroid injections may be used to minimize postoperative contracture.

To avoid inferior deviation of the lower eyelid, the lower eyelid is massaged while being pushed superiorly. This is repeated as often as tolerated, up to 30 times a day.

A common postoperative complication is dry eye syndrome.

Dry eye syndrome and chemosis

Dry eye syndrome can be caused by either insufficient tear production or excessive evaporation. The resulting lack of lubrication on the anterior surface of the eye can raise significant disruptions in activities of daily living, work, reading, computer use, and nighttime driving. Chemosis tends to accompany dry eye syndrome because both are caused by the similar etiology and requires similar treatments. Chemosis has several causative mechanisms. It can be caused by traumatic dissection, electrocautery, lymphatic dysfunction, inflammation, or postoperative lagophthalmos.

Causes of insufficient tear production include tobacco use, menopause, thyroid imbalance, medications, and aging. Schirmer's test is a method of evaluating tear production. In normal physiologic condition, the test strip will show 15-30 mm of capillary action. Less than 10 mm of capillary action demonstrates insufficient tear production. Clinically, the test is not as relevant as most cases of dry eye syndrome is caused by tear film disruption, tear distribution, or excessive evaporation.

Symptoms of dry eye syndrome and chemosis include foreign body, ocular pain, ocular fatigue, excessive tearing, light sensitivity, decreased visual acuity, and blurred vision. One significant operative cause is lagophthalmos. The eyelids do not complete cover the globe closed or blinking, with the upper and lower eyelids never coming together. Lagophthalmos after an extensive lower blepharoplasty can cause transient paralysis of the pretarsal orbicularis muscle, which improves with time. Ectropion can cause keratinization at the orifice of meibomian gland and prevents deposition onto the tear film, which causes rapid evaporation of aqueous tear without the lipid layer. This process can be reversed with correction of ectropion. A canthopexy that is too tight can also disrupt the flow of tear. In contrast, excessive excision of the skin or orbicularis oculi muscle can cause permanent disruption – especially if the pretarsal muscle is excised. Dry eye syndrome is also possible with conjunctival incision and postoperative inflammation.

Preoperatively, patients should be screened for potential risk factors such as multiple prior blepharoplasty operations, menopause, hypo/hyperthyroidism, history of dry eye syndrome, use of antihistamine, and corneal operations such as LASIK (corneal denervation).

Preventive efforts are the same for dry eye syndrome and chemosis. To allow the eyelids to close completely, the pretarsal orbicularis must be preserved, as well as the lower eyelid skin. Canthal anchoring and/or orbicularis muscle suspensions must be made secure.

Problems arising from transient exposure of the orbital globe are prevented by the application of temporary tarsorrhaphies, Frost suture, night taping of eyelids, and/or the use of eye patch. When using the eye patch, the padding must include multiple layers of gauze. Conjunctivotomy can be helpful for severe chemosis.

Medically, preoperative intravenous injection of dexamethasone (8 mg) can decrease inflammatory response. Cold compress is applied for 1 week with head elevated at all times. Because of the transient decrease in tear production, ointment containing dexamethasone and neosynephrine is used as an ointment to serve as a lubricant. Artificial tear should be instilled frequently. Dexamethasone is applied 3-4 times a day but should not be used for more than 2 weeks. It is contraindicated in patients with glaucoma. Postoperative dexamethasone is injected intramuscularly (4mg per day x 2 days). Prednisolone is an alternative and is administered over 4 days (decreasing daily doses: 40 mg, 30 mg, 20 mg, and 10 mg).

Lower blepharoplasty requires a myriad of techniques for variety of situations. Lagophthalmos is a real problem for patients with lower lid laxity and should be addressed with precise and accurate execution of procedures. To minimize complications and maximize positive outcomes, the operator must have complete understanding of the anatomy of the lower eyelid and the midface as well as thorough comprehension of even the minutest details of lower blepharoplasty techniques.

Correction of lower lid lagophthalmos

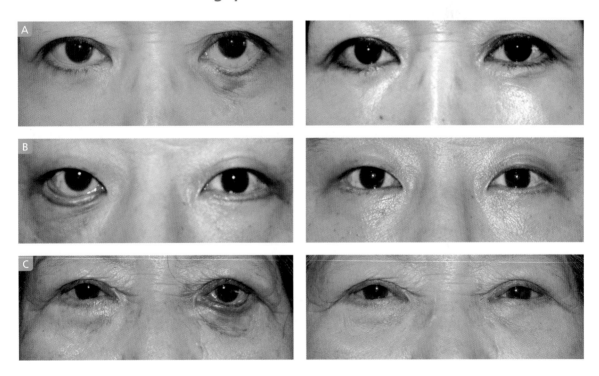

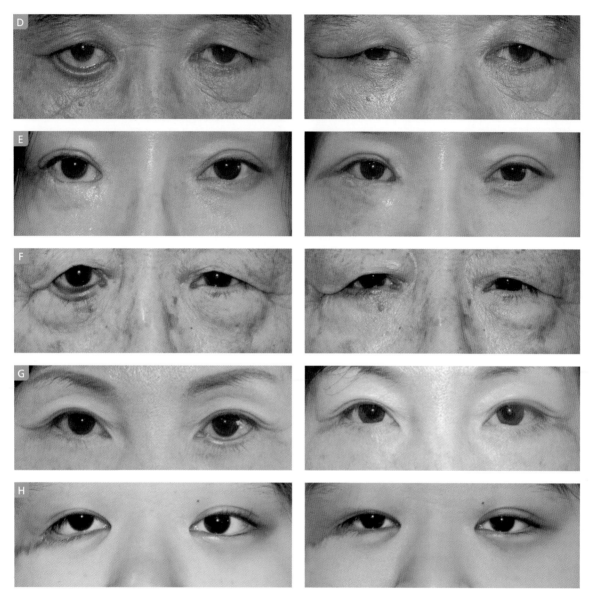

FIGURE 6-51 • Before and after correction of postoperative lagophthalmos, ectropion.

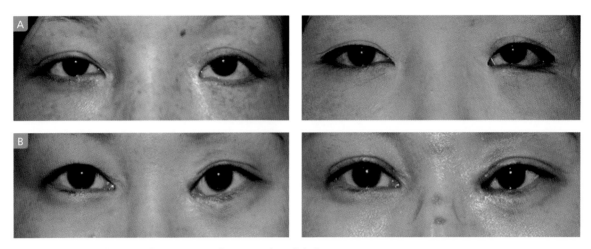

FIGURE 6-52 • Before and after correction of traumatic lagophthalmos.

COMPLICATIONS OF LATERAL CANTHOPLASTY

Types of complication (FIGURE 6-53)

- Mucosal exposure
- Lower eyelid malposition: ectropion, scleral show, and distraction
- Negative canthal tilt
- Unnatural lower eyelid curvature, lateral bowing
- Wide lateral scleral triangle
- Conjunctival injection, conjunctival web
- Entropion

Correction techniques

- V-Y advancement
- Canthal anchoring
- OOM suspension
- Spacer graft
- Epilation

Whereas most complications of epicanthoplasty represent technical failures,

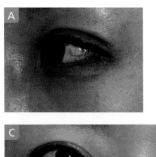
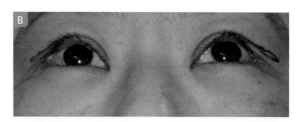
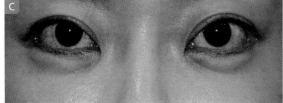
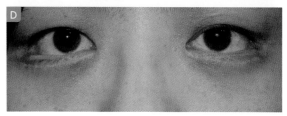
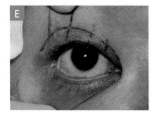

FIGURE 6-53 • Complications of lateral canthoplasty.
A. Mucosal exposure. **B.** Entropion. **C.** Scleral show and negatie canthal tilt. **D.** Ectropion, scleral show, and negative canthal tilt. **E.** Conjunctival webbing.

However, complications of lateral canthoplasty have congenital basis. Epincanthoplasty uncovers the skin covering the lacrimal caruncle. In constrast, lateral canthoplasty requires horizontal incision and extension of the lower eyelid. This extended portion of the eyelid contains neither eyelashes nor grey line. Because of this, patients must understand all of the potential pitfalls and complications of lateral canthoplasty before an operation.

Plastic surgery is a creative discipline with a basis in physiology. In contrast, surgical manipulation of the human body with no regard for its natural working order is a destructive process. The operator must be careful not to compromise with vain desires.

In lateral canthoplasty, one thing to keep in mind is that any procedure that weakens the lateral canthus should be avoided because such procedure would accelerate the process of aging. Lateral bowing is also a type of aging phenomenon and should be considered.

Complications after lateral canthoplasty includes uncomplicated mucosal exposure and various lid malposition. Mucosal exposure can be adequately addressed with excision and closure or with V-Y advancement **(FIGURE 6-54)**. However, the wide variety of malposition requires the techniques mentioned for lower blepharoplasty.

For lower blepharoplasty, canthal anchoring (canthopexy, canthoplasty) is essential with orbicularis oculi muscle being supplementary. Retraction resulting from posterior lamella contraction may require spacer graft (FIGURE 6-55). Overcorrection may be required depending on the symptoms. For example, severe negative canthal tilt requires that the lateral canthus be fixated high. If the lower eyelid does not oppose the globe with adequate tension, the canthoplasty should be secured deep in the orbital wall.

Correction of simple mucosal exposure

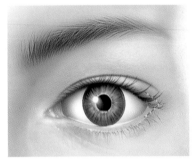 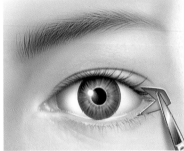 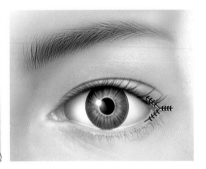

FIGURE 6-54 • Correction of mucosal exposure using V-Y advancement.

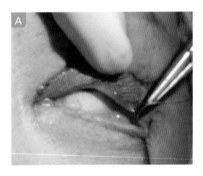 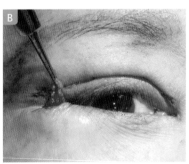

FIGURE 6-55 • Lower lid malposition as a complication of lateral canthoplasty. **A.** Canthopexy. **B.** Orbicularis oculi muscle suspension.

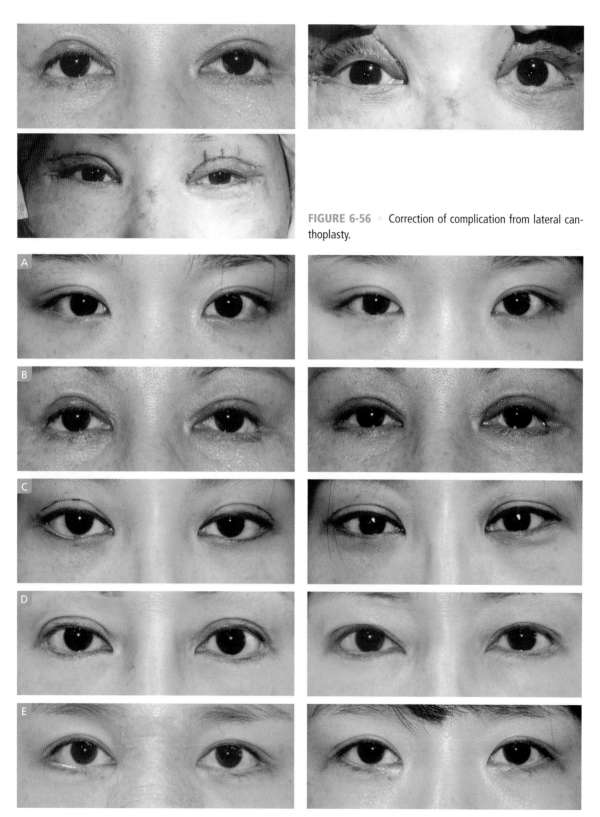

FIGURE 6-56 Correction of complication from lateral canthoplasty.

FIGURE 6-57 Correction of various canthoplasty complications.
A. Ectropion. **B.** Negative canthal tilt. **C, D.** Scleral show. **E.** Lid distraction.

LOWER EYELID ENTROPION

Entropion of the lower eyelid allows the eyelashes to come into contact with the cornea. Etiology of entropion can be divided:

- Congenital: Primary entropion and entropion secondary to epicanthus and epiblepharon
- Acquired: Involutional and cicatrical entropion

Common complications after entropion correction

- Recurrence of entropion
- Scar: long incisional scar and depressed scar
- Lower eyelid crease
- Scleral show
- Pretarsal flatness

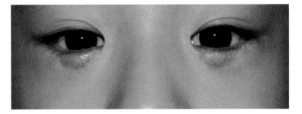

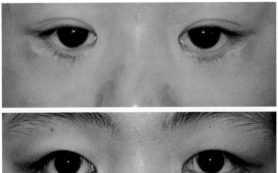

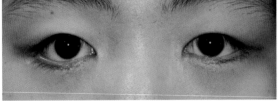

FIGURE 6-58 ● Scleral show after correction of entropion. Before and after operation photograph.

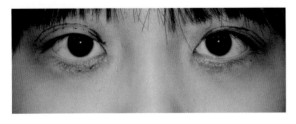

FIGURE 6-59 ● Depressed scar and lack of pretarsal fullness. Before and after operation photograph.

Corrective methods for entropion

- Lower eyelid incision
- Division of orbicularis muscle and exposure of tarsal plate
- Fixation of orbicularis muscle in the upper flap to the lower border of tarsal plate or to retractor
- Electrocautery of hair follicles
- Excision of orbicularis muscle and skin

The skin is incised 2 mm inferior to the eyelashes. In congenital forms, entropion is severe towards the central and medial areas with relatively unaffected lateral eyelid. The orbicularis oculi muscle is divided, and the tarsal plate is exposed. Next, the orbicularis muscle is fixated to the lower border of the tarsal plate, or if the entropion is severe, the muscle is fixated to the capsulopalpebral fascia **(FIGURE 6-60A, B)**. In the most severe cases, a hatch incision is made in the tarsal plate to allow the plate to bend. If the entropion cannot be corrected by any other means especially in the medial corner , the hair follicles are cauterized.

In the presence of severe epicanthal fold or epiblepharon, the skin and orbicularis muscle can be excised. The common misconception is that the skin has to be excised along with the orbicularis muscle. However, excision of orbicularis muscle should be avoided except in the case of orbicularis hypertrophy. Excision of orbicularis muscle is to be avoided because it can lead to functional problems (tear pump,

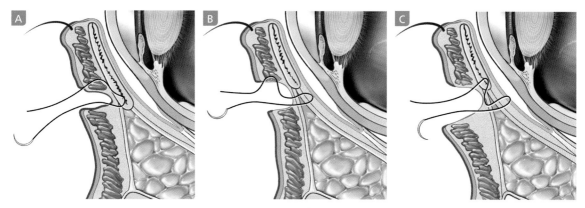

FIGURE 6-60 • **A.** Correction of entropion. The orbicularis oculi muscle is fixed to the lower portion of tarsal plate. **B.** For severe entropion, the orbicularis oculi muscle is fixated to the capsulopalpebral fascia. **C.** Reverse ptosis operation. The lower portion of tarsal plate is fixated to the capsulopalpebral fascia.

lower eyelid position and laxity, blinking) as well as aesthetic problems (pretarsal fullness).

Acquired entropion from degenerative change is caused by dehiscence of the retractor (capsulopalpebral fascia). In such cases, the orbicularis oculi muscle and tarsal plate is separated, and the retractor is fixated to the upper portion of the tarsal plate. Additionally, if the lower eyelid margin covers much of the lower limbus (reverse ptosis), the lower border of tarsus is fixed to the retractor, which can lower the eyelid margin without causing ectropion.

The difference between correction of reverse ptosis and correction of entropion is that the capsulopalpebral fascia is fixated to the lower portion of the tarsal plate for reverse ptosis. The correction of entropion can be likened to hinge door, whereas the correction of reverse ptosis is like sliding door (FIGURE 6-60C).

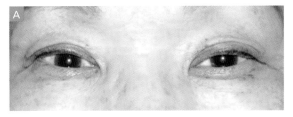
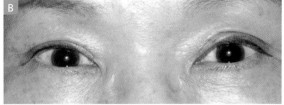

FIGURE 6-61 • Before and after reverse ptosis operation.

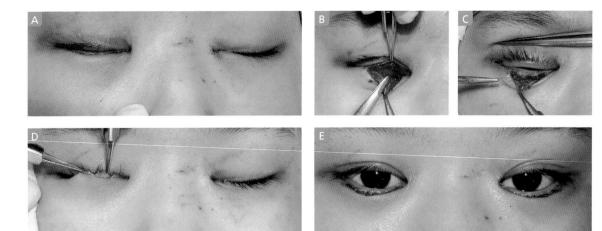

FIGURE 6-62 • A. Skin incision. The lateral portion of eyelid margin is not involved and is spared from incision. B. The orbicularis muscle is fixated to the lower portion of tarsal plate. C. After 4-5 fixations, the lower eyelid is more out-turned. D. Excision of redundant skin. E. Immediate postoperative photograph.

Summary of techniques

- Congenital entropion: orbicularis oculi muscle to the lower portion of tarsal plate
- Acquired entropion: the capsulopalpebral fascia to upper portion of tarsal plate
- Reverse ptosis: the capsulopalpebral fascia to lower portion of tarsal plate

Post-blepharoplasty canthal webbing

In this complication, the upper and lower eyelid margins are fused after lower blepharoplasty. Patients often complain decreased size of palpebral fissure as well as difficulty in opening the eyes wide.

Etiology

At the time of blepharoplasty, the lateral extension of the incision should have a smooth curve. When this transition is abrupt (angled), the skin excision can be uneven along the length of the eyelid margin, with more skin being taken away at

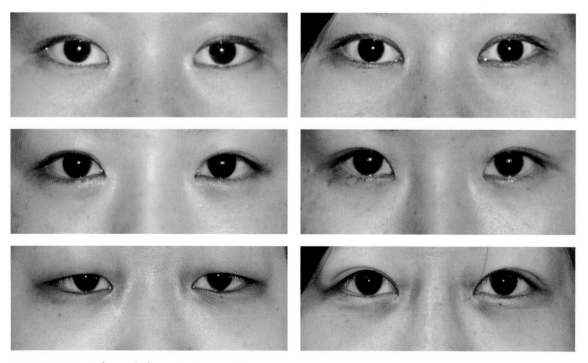

FIGURE 6-63 • Before and after entropion correction.

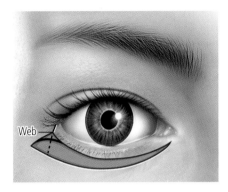

FIGURE 6-64 • Etiology of canthal webbing.
The webbing occurs where the tension is greatest after skin closure. This can be avoided by making sure that the lateral extension is made at an obtuse angle without abrupt angular changes.

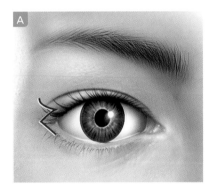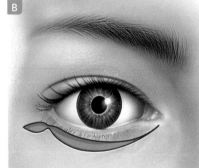

FIGURE 6-65 • Correction of canthal webbing.
A. The Z-plasty design for web correction. **B.** During lower blepharoplasty, more of the skin is preserved in the area of insufficiency.

the lateral portion. This increases the tension near the canthus, which causes the webbing **(FIGURE 6-64)**.

Correction of canthal webbing

Z-plasty (FIGURE 6-65A)

The main incision of Z-plasty is made along the webbing itself. The lower limb of Z-plasty is made along the prior incision, and the upper limb begins at the top end of the webbing and should be parallel to the lower eyelid incision. The contracture is released, and the two triangular flaps are interposed.

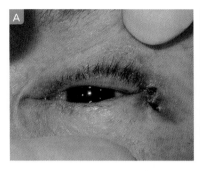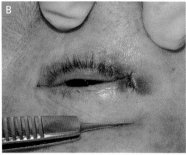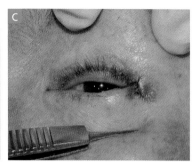

FIGURE 6-66 • Correction of canthal webbing.
A. Z-plasty design. **B.** Incision and dissection. **C.** Flap interposition and closure.

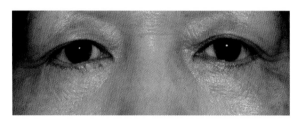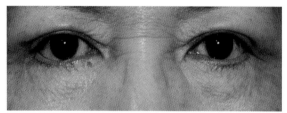

FIGURE 6-67 • Before and after correction of webbing.

Redo blepharoplasty

The skin is excised in such a manner that preserves the skin at the prior site of canthal webbing, which minimizes isolated tension at the site.

📄 REFERENCES

1. McCord CD, Ford DT, Hanna K, Hester TR, Codner MA, Nahai F : Lateral canthal anchoring : Special Situations. Plast Reconstr Surg 116:1149, 2005.
2. Patipa M : The evaluation and management of lower eyelid retraction following cosmetic surgery. Plast Reconstr Surg 106:438, 2000.
3. Park J, Putterman AM : Revisional eyelid surgery : Treatment of severe postblepharoplasty lower eyelid retraction. Facial Plastic Surgery Clinics of North America 561, 2005.
4. Lee EJ : Midface lifting through subcilliary incision. J Korean Soc Plast Reconstr 105:204, 1999.
5. Sullivan SA, Daily RA : Graft contraction : A comparision of acellular dermis versus lid hard palate mucosa in lower eyelid surgery. Ophalmic Plast Reconstr Surg 19(1):14, 2003.
6. Taban M, Douglas R, Li T, Goldberg RA, Shorr N. Efficacy of "thick" acellular human dermis (AlloDerm) for lower eyelid reconstruction: comparison with hard palate and thin AlloDerm grafts. Arch Facisl Plast surg 7:38, 2005.
7. Honig JF : Subperiosteal endotine assisted vertical upper midface lift. Aesthetic Surg J 27:276, 2007.
8. Hamra ST : Septal reset in midface rejuvenation. Aesthetic Surg J 25:628, 2005.
9. Fagien S : Reducing the incidence of dry eye symptoms after blepharoplasty. Aesthetic Surg J 24:464-8, 2004.
10. Haddock NT, Saadeh PB, Boutros S, Thorne CH. The tear trough and lid/cheek junction: anatomy and implication for surgical correction. Plast Reconst Surg 123:1332, 2009.

Index

Index